The Primary FRCA Structured Oral Examination Study Guide 1

LARA WIJAYASIRI MBBS BSc FRCA
Specialist Registrar Anaesthetics
St George's Hospital, London

KATE McCOMBE MBBS MRCP FRCA
Specialist Registrar Anaesthetics
Poole Hospital, Dorset

and

AMISH PATEL MBBS FRCA
Consultant, Intensive Care Medicine & Anaesthetics
The Royal Surrey County Hospital, Guildford

Foreword by

DAVID BOGOD
Consultant Anaesthetist
Editor-in-Chief, Anaesthesia

Radcliffe Publishing
Oxford • New York

Radcliffe Publishing Ltd
St Marks House
Shepherdess Walk
London
N1 7BQ

www.radcliffe-oxford.com

Electronic catalogue and worldwide online ordering facility.

British Library Cataloguing in Publication Data

A catalogue record for this book is available from the British Library.

ISBN-13: 978 184619 270 8

The paper used for the text pages of this book
is FSC certified. FSC (The Forest Stewardship
Council) is an international network to promote
responsible management of the world's forests.

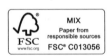

MIX
Paper from
responsible sources
FSC® C013056

Typeset by Pindar NZ, Auckland, New Zealand
Printed and bound by TJI Digital, Padstow, Cornwall, UK

Contents

Foreword

Whatever happened to the Senior Registrar? When I was a first-year trainee, we knew where to go for help, whether with a difficult case, an obstreperous colleague or an upcoming exam. The consultants were too remote and, more importantly, not always in possession of the latest facts. The SR, omnipresent and omnipotent, was a god-like creature; men wanted to be like them, women wanted to bear their children. A study published when I was in my second year of training showed that anaesthetic SRs had the lowest rate of critical incidents of any grade of anaesthetists, despite looking after the sickest patients; none of my SHO colleagues was in the least bit surprised.

While the title may have passed into history, the spirit of the Senior Registrar is alive and kicking in the forms of Drs McCombe, Wijayasiri and Patel (although Dr Patel has now made it to the top). They all passed their FRCA Primary first time and then – having ticked off the rest of the exam in a similarly airy fashion – immediately settled down to help others do the same. This book is the result.

What sets this book apart from others purporting to smooth your passage through the Primary? The authors have paid scrupulous attention to the Royal College's guide to the exam, covering not only the topics listed in the current edition, but also those in the previous edition, many of which still come up in the Structured Oral Examination (SOE). Rather than cherry-picking a number of topics from the long College syllabus, they have dealt with each and every one of them, from as many different angles as they could imagine the examiners finding.

As well as using this scrupulously comprehensive approach, the authors have included vignettes on those critical incidents such as blood transfusion error and local anaesthetic toxicity (*Study Guide 2*) which are likely to form part of the clinical SOE. A section on 'special patient groups' (*Study Guide 2*) covers topics such as diabetes, neonates, Jehovah's Witnesses and obese patients, in a format which allows the candidate to easily incorporate the information into problems posed during the SOE. The pharmacology section (*Study Guide 2*) includes 'spider diagrams' for all commonly used drugs in anaesthesia; the consistency of this unique format makes it easier to find and absorb information quickly in those angina-inducing hours before the MCQ or SOE. The 'physics' section (*Study Guide 1*) covers all those topics which the consultants have either long-forgotten or – perhaps even worse – have made their pet interest upon which they can expound throughout a long plastics list. Here, everything is handled in a page or two of short notes; information-rich and waffle-poor, these short vignettes are just what are needed as the exam date looms nearer.

In short, if you are not lucky enough to be working in the same hospital as the authors, and can't approach them for exam practice (or even if you can), then this book is an essential companion and a true *vade mecum*. Look it up – a bit of Latin can still impress the examiners!

David Bogod
Consultant Anaesthetist, Nottingham
Editor-in-Chief, *Anaesthesia*
January 2010

Preface

During our revision for the primary exam we were advised that the best way to ensure success in the structured oral examination (SOE) was to prepare answers to all of the questions in the back of *The Royal College of Anaesthetists Guide to the FRCA Examination, The Primary*. Undoubtedly, this was excellent advice but it proved an enormous task and one we simply did not have time to complete before our own exams. However, once they were over, we began to answer all those questions in the hope that this might help others to prepare for the Primary, or for the basic science component of the Final FRCA. Finally, then, here is the result: the book we wish we'd had.

The Primary FRCA Structured Oral Examination Study Guide provides answers to the questions regularly posed by the examiners. We have not attempted to write the next great anaesthetic textbook, but rather to collate information and deliver it in a relevant and user-friendly layout to make your exam preparation a little easier.

In the SOE itself, each topic will be examined for approximately five minutes. Many of these answers contain much more information than could reasonably be expected of you in that time; however, we have tried to cover several angles of questioning.

We have included the usual chapters on physiology, physics (*Study Guide 1*) and pharmacology (*Study Guide 2*) and, in addition, have written a section on patients who present the anaesthetist with unique problems, 'special patient groups' (*Study Guide 2*). These patients tend to appear in the clinical SOE before some terrible 'critical incident' befalls them. Again, we have included a section addressing the 'critical incidents' beloved of the examiner, with advice as to how to approach them in the SOE (*Study Guide 2*).

There is a unique pharmacology section including information on drugs commonly examined presented in a spider diagram layout. These extremely visual learning aids allowed us to revise the drugs in the necessary detail, and helped us to recall the information even under the acute stress of the exam. We hope you find them just as useful.

We wish you every success in what is undoubtedly a rigorous exam. We believe the key to this success is to practise presenting the knowledge that you already have, logically and concisely. The only way to do this is to practise speaking, even though the possibility of exposing any ignorance is daunting. The more you talk, the more you will cover, and every question is so much easier to answer in the exam if you have already had a dress rehearsal. We hope this book will help you in your preparations.

Good luck!

Lara Wijayasiri
Kate McCombe
Amish Patel
January 2010

'Examinations are formidable even to the best prepared,
for the greatest fool may ask more than the wisest man can answer.'

CC Colton

To Andrew, who makes me believe anything is possible.
Kate McCombe

To Amish, my husband and best friend, thank you
for helping me achieve this.
Lara Wijayasiri

To Lara, my wife and soul mate.
Amish Patel

Contributors

Dr Barbara Lattuca MBBCh MRCP FRCA
Specialist Registrar Anaesthetics
St George's Hospital, London

Physiology
- Acid–base balance
- Buffers
- Renal blood flow
- Renal handling of glucose, sodium and inulin
- Fluid compartments
- Osmoregulation
- Pain pathways

Dr Mark Wyldbore MBBS BSc(Hons) RAMC
ST4 Anaesthetics
St George's Hospital, London

Physiology
- Reflexes

Physics
- General aspects of pressure
- Pressure regulators
- Electrical components
- Defibrillators
- Electrical safety
- Diathermy

The Primary FRCA Examination

The Primary FRCA is divided into two parts; a Multiple Choice Question (MCQ) paper followed by an Objective Structured Clinical Exam (OSCE) and a Structured Oral Examination (SOE). The MCQ paper takes place on one day (at various locations throughout the UK) and some weeks later the OSCE and SOE take place together at the Royal College of Anaesthetists in London. There are three exam sittings per year.

GENERAL GUIDELINES

MCQ

➤ You are allowed a maximum of five attempts at the MCQ examination (this also applies to those candidates who have failed the examination under previous eligibility criteria).
➤ The MCQ paper must be passed in order to progress to the OSCE and SOE.

OSCE and SOE

➤ The OSCE and SOE are now marked as stand-alone examinations.
➤ At the first attempt, the OSCE and SOE must be taken at the same sitting. If you pass one component but fail the other, you have only to re-take the failed component. However, if you fail both components, you must continue taking them together until you have passed either one or both. You may attempt each part of the examination no more than four times.

EXAMINATION AND MARKING STRUCTURE

MCQ (3 hours)

➤ The paper consists of 90 questions covering three subsections: approximately 30 questions on pharmacology, 30 on physiology and 30 questions on physics and clinical measurement (including statistics and data interpretation).
➤ One mark is allocated for each correct answer.
➤ The paper is positively marked.
➤ The pass mark is expected to be approximately 80%.
➤ Your performance in each of the three subsections is taken into consideration; those who perform very poorly in one or more subsections will fail the MCQ regardless of a cumulative mark higher than the pass mark.
➤ The single best answer (SBA) format for some questions will be introduced from 2011.

OSCE (1 hour 50 minutes)

➤ The OSCE consists of 18 stations, of which only 16 are counted towards your examination score.
➤ Two 'trial stations' are included in the 18 in order to test new questions, but neither

the examiners nor the candidates will know which stations these are. The results of these two will not contribute towards your final mark.

➤ The stations comprise resuscitation, technical skills, anatomy (which may include a general procedure), history taking, physical examination, communication skills, X-ray interpretation, anaesthetic equipment, monitoring equipment, measuring equipment and anaesthetic hazards.

➤ Some stations may involve the use of a simulator.

➤ Each station is marked out of 20, with the pass mark for each station being predetermined by the examiners by modified Angoff referencing.

➤ Your aggregate score (the sum of the marks obtained at each station) will be calculated and either a 'pass' or 'fail' awarded depending on your overall performance.

SOE 1 (30 minutes)

➤ Two examiners conduct each SOE. You will be questioned by the first examiner on one subject for 15 minutes, while the other observes and marks your performance. The examiners then trade places and the previously silent one examines the second subject, while his or her partner observes.

➤ In each 15 minutes, you will be asked questions on three different topics, relating to the subject being examined. In SOE 1, these subjects are pharmacology and physiology and biochemistry.

➤ A score of 0, 1 or 2 (fail, borderline or pass) will be allocated per question by each examiner. This means that the maximum total score for SOE 1 is 24 (there are two examiners, each marking a total of six questions, each of which can receive a maximum mark of two).

SOE 2 (30 minutes)

➤ The format of SOE 2 is as described above.

➤ 15 minutes will be spent asking three questions on physics, clinical measurement, equipment and safety and the other 15 asking three questions on clinical topics, including a problem-based scenario (critical incident).

➤ The marking of SOE 2 is identical to that of SOE 1.

➤ The marks achieved for both SOE 1 and SOE 2 are combined together to give an aggregate score. The maximum total score achievable is 48. The candidate will need a score of 37 or more in order to pass.

For up-to-date information on the examination format and syllabus, visit the Royal College website: www.rcoa.ac.uk.

1

Physiology

CHAPTER 1

Haemoglobin

Why is haemoglobin essential?

Oxygen is relatively insoluble in water and therefore only approximately 1.5% of total oxygen is carried dissolved in the plasma. The remaining 98.5% is bound to haemoglobin. Haemoglobin increases the oxygen-carrying capacity of blood approximately 70-fold.

Describe the molecular structure of haemoglobin

The haemoglobin molecule consists of four porphyrin rings in association with central iron moieties (haem), each attached to a polypeptide chain (globin).

Different forms of haemoglobin exist depending on the structure of these polypeptide chains. In normal adults 98% of all haemoglobin is in the form of HbA1 (2 α chains and 2 β chains). The remaining 2% is in the form of HbA2 (2 α chains and 2 γ chains). Fetal haemoglobin (HbF) is comprised of 2 α chains and 2 γ chains. HbF changes to HbA at around 6 months of life.

What happens to haemoglobin in sickle cell anaemia?

In sickle cell disease there is an abnormal β polypeptide chain due to a genetic mutation in the amino acid sequence where the amino acid valine is replaced by glutamic acid. In the heterozygous state this confers an advantage against malaria as the shortened lifespan of the erythrocyte prevents the blood-borne phase of the mosquito from completing its life cycle. In the homozygous state the abnormal haemoglobin is susceptible to forming solid non-pliable sickle-like structures when exposed to low P_aO_2, causing the erythrocytes to obstruct the microcirculation, leading to painful crises and infarcts.

What happens to haemoglobin in thalassaemia?

Thalassaemia is an inherited autosomal recessive blood disease. In thalassaemia the genetic defect results in a reduced rate of synthesis of one of the globin chains that make up haemoglobin. Reduced synthesis of one of the globin chains can result in the formation of abnormal haemoglobin molecules, causing anaemia.

Thalassaemia is a quantitative problem of too few globin chains synthesised, whereas sickle cell anaemia is a qualitative problem of synthesis of an incorrectly functioning globin. Thalassaemia may thus be α or β depending on which globin chain is being underproduced.

How does oxygen bind to haemoglobin?

Oxygen binds to the ferrous iron (Fe^{2+}) in haemoglobin by forming a reversible bond. There is no oxidative reaction and so the iron atom always remains in the ferrous form. In the condition methaemoglobinaemia, the ferrous iron is oxidised into the ferric (Fe^{3+}) form.

Each molecule of haemoglobin can bind four molecules of oxygen (i.e. one at each ferrous ion within each haem group). There are several factors that influence binding including local oxygen tension, local tissue environment (temperature, CO_2, hydrogen ions and 2,3 DPG) and the allosteric change and cooperative binding behaviour of oxygen to haemoglobin (see oxygen–haemoglobin dissociation curve question, Chapter 2, for further details).

Can the dissolved fraction of oxygen be dismissed?

Even though dissolved oxygen represents a small fraction of total oxygen-carrying capacity of the blood it still constitutes an important fraction. Severe anaemia illustrates the point, e.g. for a Jehovah's Witness who has experienced a massive intraoperative haemorrhage and refuses blood transfusion, one therapeutic option would be the use of hyperbaric oxygen therapy; at 3 atmospheres and using 100% oxygen the dissolved fraction of oxygen would meet total body oxygen requirements.

The dissolved fraction of oxygen is also responsible for triggering the hypoxic respiratory drive. This is of clinical significance in patients with COPD who are chronic CO_2 retainers, as giving them high flow oxygen to increase their PaO_2 may lead to loss of their hypoxic drive.

CHAPTER 2

Oxygen–haemoglobin dissociation curve

Draw the oxygen–haemoglobin dissociation curve (OHDC).
The OHDC is a graph relating the percentage of haemoglobin saturated with oxygen to the partial pressure of oxygen (PO_2).

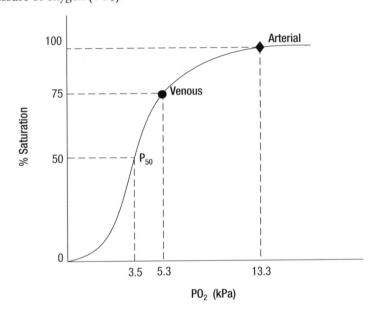

GRAPH 1.1 The oxygen–haemoglobin dissociation curve

Normal oxyhaemoglobin dissociation curve
➤ Arterial PO_2 is 13.3 kPa with a Hb saturation of 97% (it is not 100% due to venous admixture constituting physiological shunt).
➤ Venous PO_2 is 5.3 kPa with a Hb saturation of 75%.
➤ P_{50} is 3.5 kPa (this is the PO_2 at which Hb is 50% saturated and it is the conventional point used to compare the oxygen affinity of Hb).

Explain the shape of the OHDC
The OHDC has a characteristic sigmoid shape due to the binding characteristics of haemoglobin to oxygen.
➤ **Allosteric modulation** – When oxygen binds to haemoglobin, the two β chains move closer together and change the position of the haem moieties which assume a 'relaxed' or R state. When oxygen dissociates from haemoglobin, the reverse happens and the haem moieties take up a 'tense' or T state.
➤ **Cooperative binding** – When oxygen binds to haemoglobin the R state is favoured, which has an increased affinity for oxygen and so facilitates the uptake of additional

7

oxygen. The affinity of haemoglobin for the fourth oxygen molecule is therefore much greater than for the first.

What are the major physiological factors that determine the position of the OHDC?
Factors that shift the OHDC to the right: this facilitates the unloading of oxygen into tissues and the P_{50} value is higher than 3.5 kPa:

➤ ↓ pH
➤ ↑ temperature
➤ ↑ 2,3-diphosphoglycerate
➤ ↑ $PaCO_2$
➤ HbS
➤ anaemia
➤ pregnancy
➤ post-acclimatisation to altitude.

Factors that shift the OHDC to the left: this facilitates the uptake of oxygen from the lungs and the P_{50} value is lower than 3.5 kPa:

➤ ↑ pH
➤ ↓ temperature
➤ ↓ 2,3-diphosphoglycerate
➤ ↓ $PaCO_2$
➤ HbF
➤ methaemoglobin
➤ carboxyhaemoglobin
➤ stored blood.

What is the Bohr effect?
This describes the right shift in the OHDC in association with increased $PaCO_2$ and hydrogen ion concentration.

What is the Double Bohr effect?
This refers to the situation in the placenta where the Bohr effect operates in both the maternal and fetal circulations. The increase in PCO_2 in the maternal intervillous sinuses assists oxygen unloading. The decrease in PCO_2 on the fetal side of the circulation assists oxygen loading. The Bohr effect facilitates the reciprocal exchange of oxygen for carbon dioxide. The Double Bohr effect means that the oxygen dissociation curves for maternal HbA and fetal HbF move apart – i.e. right shift (maternal); left shift (fetal).

What is the Haldane effect?
This describes the increased ability of deoxygenated haemoglobin to carry carbon dioxide. Conversely, oxygenated blood has a reduced capacity to carry carbon dioxide. The Haldane effect occurs because deoxygenated haemoglobin is a better proton acceptor than oxyhaemoglobin.

How does the OHDC compare with the myoglobin dissociation curve?
➤ Myoglobin is an oxygen-carrying protein found in skeletal muscles (it gives muscle its dark red appearance).
➤ It consists of a single polypeptide chain associated with a haem moiety.
➤ Unlike haemoglobin, it can only bind one molecule of oxygen and therefore its dissociation curve is a rectangular hyperbola.
➤ Myoglobin also has a higher affinity for oxygen than haemoglobin and so its dissociation curve lies to the left of the OHDC.

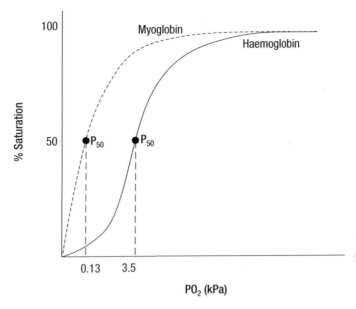

GRAPH 1.2 Myoglobin dissociation curve compared to oxyhaemoglobin dissociation curve

➤ Myoglobin takes up oxygen from the circulating haemoglobin and releases it into exercising muscle tissues at very low PO_2, thus providing a source of oxygen during periods of sustained muscle contractions when blood flow to these muscles may be constricted due to blood vessel compression.

CHAPTER 3

Hypoxia

Hypoxia is a core respiratory physiology question and as such examiners will expect a thorough understanding of this topic. Structure your answer.

Define hypoxia and classify the causes

Hypoxia may be defined either as an inadequate oxygen supply, or the inability to utilise oxygen at a cellular level. Causes are divided into four main types:

➤ **Hypoxic hypoxia** – an arterial PaO_2 < 12 kPa
  - Low FiO_2, e.g. inadvertent hypoxic gas delivery during anaesthesia
  - Hypoventilation, e.g. opiate-induced
  - Diffusion impairment, e.g. pulmonary oedema, pulmonary fibrosis
  - Ventilation-perfusion mismatch, e.g. COPD, asthma, LRTI
  - Shunt, e.g. atelectasis causing intrapulmonary shunt

➤ **Anaemic hypoxia** – normal PaO_2 but inadequate oxygen-carrying capacity
  - Low circulating haemoglobin level, e.g. acute and chronic anaemias
  - Normal circulating haemoglobin level but reduced ability to carry oxygen, e.g. carbon monoxide poisoning

➤ **Stagnant hypoxia** – normal PaO_2 and oxygen-carrying capacity but reduced tissue and organ perfusion
  - e.g. cardiogenic shock

➤ **Histotoxic hypoxia** – normal PaO_2, oxygen-carrying capacity and tissue perfusion but an inability of the tissues to utilise the oxygen at a cellular mitochondrial level
  - e.g. cyanide poisoning

Draw oxyhaemoglobin dissociation curves for saturation showing arterial ♦; and mixed venous •; points in the four types of hypoxia

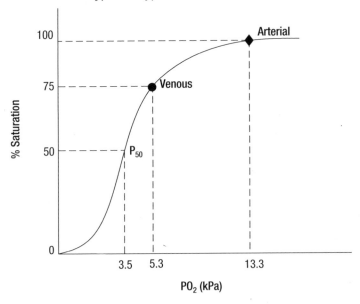

GRAPH 1.3 Normal oxyhaemoglobin dissociation curve

➤ Arterial PaO_2 13.3 kPa.
➤ Venous PO_2 5.3 kPa.
➤ P_{50} 3.5 kPa (partial pressure of oxygen at which haemoglobin is 50% saturated).

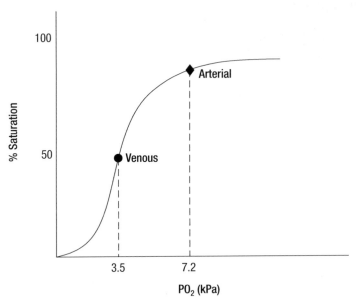

GRAPH 1.4 Oxyhaemoglobin dissociation curve in hypoxic hypoxia

➤ Arterial PaO_2 is reduced.
➤ Venous desaturation (<75%).

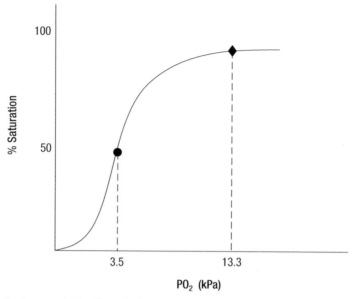

GRAPH 1.5 Oxyhaemoglobin dissociation curve in anaemic hypoxia

➤ Arterial PaO_2 remains normal (>13.3 kPa).
➤ However, global oxygen delivery is reduced from anaemia/reduced oxygen content.
➤ Result is increased oxygen extraction and venous desaturation.

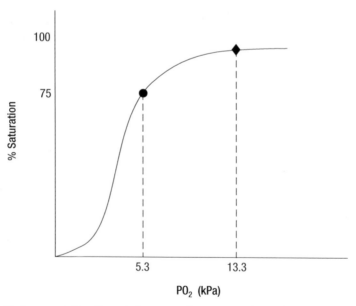

GRAPH 1.6 Oxyhaemoglobin dissociation curve in stagnant hypoxia

➤ Arterial PaO_2 is normal.
➤ Venous PO_2 is normal.
➤ Tissues/organs do not receive the oxygenated blood due to perfusion failure.

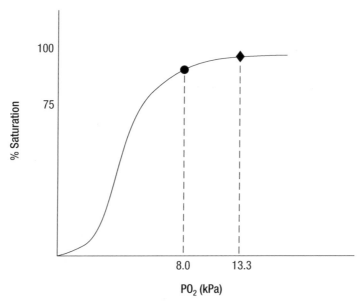

GRAPH 1.7 Oxyhaemoglobin dissociation curve in histotoxic hypoxia

➤ Arterial PaO_2 is normal.
➤ Cells are unable to utilise oxygen resulting in high venous saturations.
➤ Cyanide poisoning will also be associated with a left shift of the oxyhaemoglobin dissociation curve.

What is oxygen content?
Oxygen is carried in the blood in two main ways: combined with haemoglobin and dissolved in the plasma. Oxygen content is calculated by combining the proportion of oxygen bound to haemoglobin with that dissolved.

$$\text{Oxygen content} = [\text{Bound Oxygen}] + [\text{Dissolved Oxygen}]$$
$$= [\text{Hb} \times 1.34 \times \text{SaO}_2] + [\text{PaO}_2 \times 0.0225]$$

Where:
Hb   Haemoglobin g/dL
1.34   Huffner's constant – each gram of haemoglobin combines with 1.34 mL of oxygen
SaO$_2$ Arterial oxygen saturation as a percentage, e.g. 96% = 0.96
PaO$_2$ Partial pressure of oxygen determines fraction of dissolved oxygen
0.0225 mL of oxygen per dL per kPa of oxygen partial pressure.

Thus oxygen content may be calculated for arterial and venous blood.
E.g. arterial oxygen content (CaO_2): Hb 15 g/dL, SaO_2 100% and PaO_2 13.3 kPa

$$\text{Arterial oxygen content} = [15 \times 1.34 \times 1.0] + [13.3 \times 0.0225]$$
$$= [20.1] + [0.3]$$
$$= 20.4 \text{ mL of oxygen per dL}$$

Venous oxygen content ($C\bar{v}O_2$) Hb 15 g/dL, SvO_2 75% and PvO_2 5.3 kPa
$$C\bar{v}O_2 = [15 \times 1.34 \times 0.75] + [5.3 \times 0.0225]$$
$$= [15] + [0.2]$$
$$= 15.2 \text{ mL of oxygen per dL}$$

Note that the difference between arterial and venous oxygen content is just under 5 mL of oxygen per dL. If oxygen content is multiplied by cardiac output, oxygen delivery is obtained.

If circulating volume for a 70 kg man is 80 mL/kg (5600 mL), this equates to an arterial oxygen content of just over 1000 mL and a venous oxygen content of approximately 750 mL.

Discuss arterial and venous oxygen content in the four types of hypoxia
➤ **Hypoxic hypoxia**
E.g. altitude: Hb 15 g/dL/SaO_2 85%/PaO_2 6.5 kPa/PvO_2 3.0 kPa/SvO_2 45%

$$CaO_2 = [15 \times 1.34 \times 0.85] + [6.5 \times 0.0225] = 17\,mL\,O_2/dL$$
$$C\bar{v}O_2 = [15 \times 1.34 \times 0.45] + [3.0 \times 0.0225] = 9\,mL\,O_2/dL$$

Note arterial oxygen content is reduced and there is increased oxygen extraction resulting in a lower venous oxygen content.

➤ **Anaemic hypoxia**
E.g. haemorrhage: Hb 7 g/dL/SaO_2 100%/PaO_2 13.3 kPa/PvO_2 4.0 kPa/SvO_2 50%

$$CaO_2 = [7 \times 1.34 \times 1.0] + [13.3 \times 0.0225] = 10\,mL\,O_2/dL$$
$$C\bar{v}O_2 = [7 \times 1.34 \times 0.5] + [4.0 \times 00225] = 5\,mL\,O_2/dL$$

Significant reduction in arterial oxygen content and hence oxygen delivery to the tissues. There will be a resultant increase in cardiac work in an attempt to maintain oxygen delivery to the tissues.

➤ **Stagnant hypoxia**
E.g. cardiogenic shock: Hb 15 g/dL/SaO_2 100%/PaO_2 13.3 kPa/PvO_2 5.3/SvO_2 75%

$$CaO_2 = [15 \times 1.34 \times 1.0] + [13.3 \times 0.0225] = 20\,mL\,O_2/dL$$
$$C\bar{v}O_2 = [15 \times 1.34 \times 0.75] + [5.3 \times 0.0225] = 15\,mL\,O_2/dL$$

Note arterial oxygen content is normal. However, circulatory dysfunction results in inadequate oxygen delivery to organs and venous saturations may even be increased.

➤ **Histotoxic hypoxia**
E.g. cyanide: Hb 15 g/dL/SaO_2 100%/PaO_2 13.3 kPa/PvO_2 8.0 kPa/SvO_2 90%

$$CaO_2 = [15 \times 1.34 \times 1.0] + [13.3 \times 0.0225] = 20\,mL\,O_2/dL$$
$$C\bar{v}O_2 = [15 \times 1.34 \times 0.9] + [8.0 \times 0.0225] = 18\,mL\,O_2/dL$$

Arterial oxygen content is normal. However, at a cellular level there is an inability to utilise oxygen, resulting in high venous oxygen content. This picture may also be seen in severe sepsis where despite adequate oxygen delivery cellular hypoxia remains with high central venous saturations.

CHAPTER 4

Oxygen transport

Oxygen transport is a fundamental respiratory physiology question and examiners will expect complete understanding of the topic.

How is oxygen transported from the lungs to the cells of the tissues?
➤ Ventilation of the lungs supplies oxygen to the alveolus.
➤ Diffusion of oxygen across the alveolus to the pulmonary capillaries.
➤ Oxygen carriage by blood (combined with haemoglobin or dissolved in plasma).
➤ Diffusion from capillary to mitochondria.

The oxygen cascade describes the sequential reduction in PO_2 from atmosphere to cellular mitochondria.
   Oxygen is present in the air at a concentration of 21%.
   Atmospheric pressure at sea level is 1 atmosphere = 101 kPa.
   This equates to an inspired oxygen concentration of 21 kPa.
   At the mitochondrial level the PO_2 is only 1–5 kPa.

Describe what occurs at each step of the oxygen cascade
➤ Inspired PO_2 at sea level is 21 kPa (atmospheric pressure × % oxygen in air).
➤ Humidification of inspired air occurs in the upper respiratory tract. The humidity is formed by water vapour, which as a gas exerts a pressure. At 37°C the saturated vapour pressure (SVP) of water in the trachea is 6.3 kPa. Taking the SVP into account, the PO_2 in the trachea when breathing air is $(101.3–6.3) × 0.21 = 19.95$ kPa.
➤ By the time the oxygen has reached the alveoli the PO_2 has fallen to about 15 kPa. This is because the PO_2 of the gas in the alveoli (P_AO_2) is a balance between two processes:

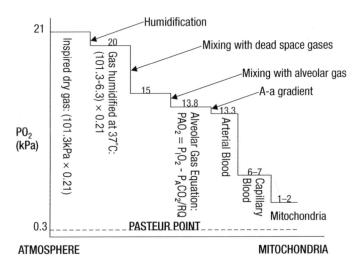

FIGURE 1.8 The oxygen cascade

the removal of oxygen by the pulmonary capillaries and its continual supply by alveolar ventilation (breathing) – thus hypoventilation will result in a lower alveolar PO_2.

➤ Blood returning to the heart from the tissues has a low PO_2 (5.3 kPa) and travels to the lungs via the pulmonary arteries. The pulmonary arteries form pulmonary capillaries, which surround the alveoli. Oxygen diffuses from the high pressure in the alveoli (15 kPa) to the area of lower pressure of the blood in the pulmonary capillaries (5.3 kPa). After oxygenation blood moves into the pulmonary veins which return to the left side of the heart to be pumped to the systemic tissues. In a 'perfect lung' the PO_2 of pulmonary venous blood would be equal to the PO_2 in the alveolus. Three factors may cause the PO_2 in the pulmonary veins to be less than the P_AO_2: ventilation/perfusion mismatch, shunt and diffusion impairment. These are the causes of an increased Alveolar–arterial (A–a) gradient.

➤ Arterial blood with a PaO_2 of 13.3 kPa passes to the tissues – the capillary PO_2 being in the order of 6–7 kPa.

➤ Oxygen then diffuses to the cells in the capillary beds, the mitochondria receiving a PO_2 of 1–5 kPa depending on the capillary bed.

➤ An increase in the size of any of the 'steps' in the oxygen cascade may result in hypoxia at the mitochondrial level.

What are the causes of an increased A–a gradient?

Under normal circumstances the A–a gradient is less than 2 kPa (P_AO_2 15 kPa / PaO_2 13.3 kPa) and is caused by small ventilation–perfusion ($\dot{V}/\dot{Q}$) mismatch and shunt present in normal healthy individuals.

However, an increased A–a gradient is present in disease states that result in an increase in $\dot{V}/\dot{Q}$ mismatch/shunt or conditions which impair diffusion.

➤ **Diffusion impairment**, e.g. pulmonary oedema or pulmonary fibrosis
➤ **$\dot{V}/\dot{Q}$ mismatch**, e.g. severe hypotension, COPD, LRTI or asthma
➤ **Shunt:**
  • intrapulmonary causes, e.g. LRTI or atelectasis
  • extrapulmonary causes, e.g. right to left cardiac shunt.

What are the causes of hypoxia? (see also Chapter 3)

➤ Low inspired oxygen
➤ Hypoventilation
➤ Anaemic
➤ Stagnant
➤ Histotoxic
➤ $\dot{V}/\dot{Q}$ mismatch
➤ Diffusion impairment
➤ Shunt

How is oxygen transported in the blood?

➤ Oxygen is carried mainly in combination with haemoglobin and also dissolved in plasma.
➤ Each gram of haemoglobin combines with 1.34 mL of oxygen (Huffner's constant)
➤ The amount of oxygen dissolved is determined by the partial pressure of oxygen.

$$
\begin{aligned}
\text{Oxygen content} \quad &= [\text{Bound Oxygen}] + [\text{Dissolved Oxygen}] \\
&= [\text{Hb} \times 1.34 \times S_aO_2] + [PaO_2 \times 0.0225]
\end{aligned}
$$

Where:

Hb   Haemoglobin g/dL

1.34   Huffner's constant – each gram of haemoglobin combines with 1.34 mL of oxygen

SaO$_2$ Arterial oxygen saturation as a percentage, e.g. 96% = 0.96

PaO$_2$ Partial pressure of oxygen determines fraction of dissolved oxygen

0.0225   mL of oxygen per dL per kPa of oxygen partial pressure.

Thus oxygen content may be calculated for arterial and venous blood

E.g. Arterial oxygen content (CaO$_2$): Hb 15 g/dL, SaO$_2$ 100% and PaO$_2$ 13.3 kPa

$$\textbf{Arterial oxygen content} = [15 \times 1.34 \times 1.0] + [13.3 \times 0.0225]$$
$$= [20.1] + [0.3]$$
$$= 20.4 \text{ mL of oxygen per dL}$$

Venous oxygen content (C$\bar{\text{v}}$O$_2$) Hb 15 g/dL, SvO$_2$ 75% and PvO$_2$ 5.3 kPa

$$C\bar{v}O_2 = [15 \times 1.34 \times 0.75] + [5.3 \times 0.0225]$$
$$= [15] + [0.2]$$
$$= 15.2 \text{ mL of oxygen per dL}$$

Note that the difference between arterial and venous oxygen content is just under 5 mL of oxygen per dL.

If oxygen content is multiplied by cardiac output (heart rate × stroke volume) then oxygen delivery (DO$_2$) is obtained:

$$DO_2 = CO \times CaO_2$$

What methods can be used to increase oxygen content and delivery?

➤ Increase arterial oxygen content (CaO$_2$).

➤ Increase cardiac output (CO).

Increase CaO$_2$

➤ Increase circulating haemoglobin concentration (blood transfusion).

➤ Maintain high oxygen saturations (supplemental oxygen).

➤ Increase dissolved oxygen by increasing partial pressure of oxygen, e.g. hyperbaric oxygen (achieving a PO$_2$ of 3 atmospheres supplies sufficient dissolved oxygen to meet oxygen demand).

Increase CO

➤ Optimise heart rate and rhythm (rate 60–90 bpm/sinus rhythm).

➤ Optimise stroke volume (preload/contractility).

➤ Maintain perfusion pressure to ensure organ oxygen delivery (afterload).

Achieve above with fluids +/– inotropes

CHAPTER 5

Carbon dioxide transport

Carbon dioxide (CO_2) (MW 44; BP $-79\,°C$; critical temperature $31\,°C$) is one of the main end products of metabolism. The body contains approximately 120 L of CO_2.

Normal CO_2 values
➤ $PiCO_2$ Inspired CO_2 0.03 kPa
➤ $PECO_2$ Expired CO_2 4 kPa
➤ $PaCO_2$ Arterial CO_2 5.3 kPa
➤ $PACO_2$ Alveolar CO_2 5.3 kPa [CO_2 content 21.9 mmol/L]
➤ $PvCO_2$ Venous CO_2 6.1 kPa [CO_2 content 23.7 mmol/L]

How is CO_2 transported from the cells to the lungs?
Under resting conditions CO_2 production in the body is approximately 200 mL/min.
    CO_2 is transported in the blood in three forms: dissolved, as carbamino compounds and as bicarbonate. The CO_2, which is formed in the cells, diffuses through the interstitial space to enter the venous circulation.
    CO_2 is carried as:
➤ **dissolved:** 5% (CO_2 is 20 times more soluble in blood than O_2)
        (Henry's Law of CO_2 solubility 0.231 mmol/L/kPa)
➤ **carbamino compounds:** 5% (with NH_2 groups on haemoglobin)
➤ **bicarbonate:** 90% (mainly in plasma).

$$\text{Carbonic anhydrase}$$
$$CO_2 + H_2O \rightleftharpoons H_2CO_3 \rightleftharpoons H^+ + HCO_3^-$$

Draw the events in the plasma and RBCs

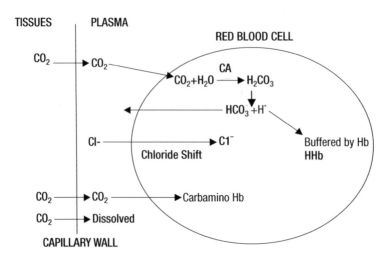

FIGURE 1.9 Schematic representation of CO_2 transport

➤ Reaction between CO_2 and H_2O is slow in the plasma but fast within the red blood cell (RBC) due to the intracellular presence of the enzyme carbonic anhydrase.
➤ HCO_3^- formed in the above reaction diffuses out of the RBC. However, the accompanying H^+ ion cannot follow due to the relative impermeability of the red cell membrane to such cations. In order to maintain electrical neutrality Cl^- ions diffuse into the red cell from the plasma, the *'chloride shift'*.
➤ Haldane effect – describes the increased capacity of deoxygenated haemoglobin to carry CO_2 compared to oxyhaemoglobin and is a result of the increased ability of deoxyhaemoglobin to bind CO_2 allowing the formation of carbamino Hb and the better buffering ability of deoxyhaemoglobin allowing more CO_2 to be transported as bicarbonate.

What events take place in the lungs?
The reverse reaction occurs whereby HCO_3^- diffuses into the red cell, accepting an H^+ ion and driving the reaction to the left forming CO_2, which can then be expired and excreted.

Compare the CO_2 dissociation curve with HbO_2 dissociation curve
➤ CO_2 dissociation curve is more linear than the oxyhaemoglobin dissociation curve.
➤ Oxyhaemoglobin carries less CO_2 than deoxyhaemoglobin for the same PCO_2 – the Haldane effect.

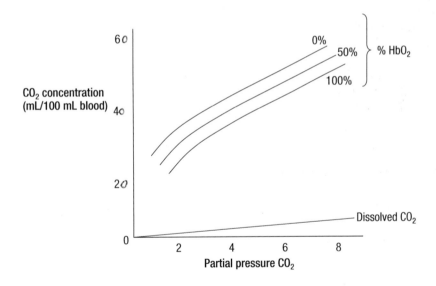

GRAPH 1.10 CO_2 dissociation curve compared to O_2 dissociation curve

Draw the physiological dissociation curve for CO_2

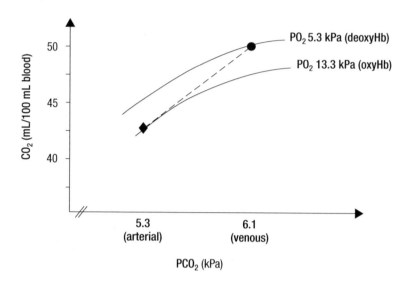

GRAPH 1.11 CO_2 dissociation curve

CHAPTER 6

Alveolar gas equation

The alveolar gas equation allows the calculation of alveolar partial pressure of oxygen for a given inspired pressure of oxygen and a given alveolar pressure of carbon dioxide.

The examiners may ask about the alveolar gas equation in various guises; ranging from a direct question such as, 'How can the partial pressure of oxygen in alveolar gas be measured?' to 'What effect would sudden decompression of a commercial aircraft at an altitude of 35 000 ft have on alveolar oxygen pressure?'

Irrespective of the format of the question it is vital to understand the key role that the alveolar gas equation plays in understanding the causes of hypoxia and ultimately understanding the alveolar–arterial oxygen difference (A–a gradient).

Alveolar gas equation:

$$P_AO_2 = PiO_2 - \frac{P_ACO_2}{R}$$

Where:

P_AO_2 Alveolar partial pressure of oxygen
PiO_2 Inspired pressure of oxygen = $FiO_2 \times (P_{ATM} - P_{H2O})$ fraction of inspired oxygen multiplied by the difference between atmospheric pressure and water vapour pressure
P_ACO_2 Alveolar partial pressure of carbon dioxide (approximates with arterial CO_2)
R Respiratory Quotient = CO_2 production/O_2 consumption (N=0.8).

Explain how PiO_2 is calculated
The inspired O_2 is different from atmospheric, because it is warmed and contains added water vapour. Fractional inspired O_2 does not vary with altitude. However, barometric pressure falls with increasing altitude – halving every 18 000 ft. Partial pressure of water vapour remains constant at 47 mmHg (6.3 kPa). Thus:

$$PiO_2 = FiO_2 \times (Patm - PH_2O)$$

E.g. At sea level (barometric pressure 760 mmHg/101 kPa)

$$PiO_2 = 0.21 \times (101 - 6.3) = 19.9 \, kPa$$

E.g. At an altitude of 63 000 ft (barometric pressure 47 mmHg/6.3 kPa)

$$PiO_2 = 0.21 \times (6.3 - 6.3) = 0$$

At 63 000 ft barometric pressure is equal to the partial pressure of water and a human being's blood would boil (as saturated vapour pressure of water would be equal to barometric pressure).

What factors affect the respiratory quotient (RQ)?
The metabolic substrates used are the main determinants of the RQ.

Carbohydrate RQ	1.0
Protein RQ	0.8–0.9
Fat RQ	0.7

Why may P_AO_2 and PaO_2 differ?
If PiO_2 is held constant and $PaCO_2$ increases, P_AO_2 and PaO_2 will always decrease. Since P_AO_2 is a calculation based on known (or assumed) factors, its change is predictable. PaO_2, by contrast, is a measurement whose theoretical maximum value is defined by P_AO_2 but whose lower limit is determined by ventilation–perfusion ($\dot{V}/\dot{Q}$) imbalance, pulmonary diffusing capacity and oxygen content of blood entering the pulmonary artery (mixed venous blood). In particular, the greater the imbalance of ventilation–perfusion ratios, the more PaO_2 tends to differ from the calculated P_AO_2. (The difference between P_AO_2 and PaO_2 is commonly referred to as the 'A–a gradient'. However, 'gradient' is a misnomer since the difference is not due to any diffusion gradient, but instead to $\dot{V}/\dot{Q}$ imbalance and/or right to left shunting of blood past ventilating alveoli. Hence 'A–a O_2 difference' is the more appropriate term.)

What is the normal A–a gradient?
The A–a gradient varies with age and FiO_2. Up to middle age, breathing ambient air, the normal A–a gradient is approximately 1.3 kPa (10 mmHg). Breathing an FiO_2 of 1.0 the normal A–a gradient ranges up to about 10 kPa. If the A–a gradient is increased above normal there is a defect of gas transfer within the lungs; this defect is almost always due to $\dot{V}/\dot{Q}$ imbalance.

What are the common causes of an increased A–a gradient?
There are three common causes:
➤ **Ventilation–perfusion ($\dot{V}/\dot{Q}$) mismatching** – Blood flowing through high $\dot{V}/\dot{Q}$ areas with a higher PO_2 cannot compensate for the blood flowing through low $\dot{V}/\dot{Q}$ areas because:
  • of the shape of the oxyhaemoglobin dissociation curve
  • more of the pulmonary blood usually flows through low $\dot{V}/\dot{Q}$ areas.
➤ **Diffusion impairment** – May occur in conditions such as pulmonary fibrosis/ pulmonary oedema. It may also occur if PiO_2 is low (e.g. high altitude) or if lung capillary transit time is greatly reduced from its normal 0.75 seconds (e.g. exercise).
➤ **Anatomical shunt** – An extreme form of $\dot{V}/\dot{Q}$ mismatch. Deoxygenated blood entering the systemic circulation.

CHAPTER 7

Ventilation–perfusion (V̇/Q̇) mismatch and shunt

Ventilation and perfusion vary across the lungs. If ventilation and perfusion are not matched the consequences for gas exchange are impairment of both O_2 uptake and CO_2 elimination.

Draw a graph to show how ventilation and perfusion are distributed across the lung

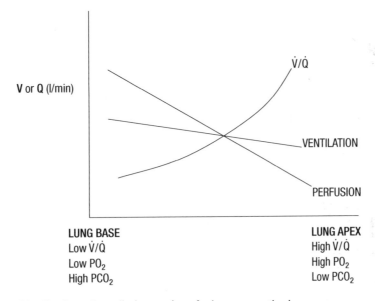

GRAPH 1.12 Distribution of ventilation and perfusion across the lung

Explain the observed differences seen in ventilation and perfusion across the lung
➤ The lungs are essentially suspended within the thoracic cavity and therefore the alveoli are subjected to the effects of gravity. Consequently, the alveoli at the lung apex are relatively larger than those at the bases.
➤ The apical alveoli are thus on a flatter part of their pressure–volume (i.e. compliance) curve than the basal alveoli, which are on the steep portion of the compliance curve.
➤ Hence, ventilation is preferentially distributed to the basal alveoli.
➤ The pulmonary circulation differs from the systemic circulation. It is a low-pressure system with a blood volume of approximately 500 mL.
➤ Gravitational forces affect pulmonary blood flow through vessel distension and recruitment and thus the bases of the lungs have higher blood flow than the apices.
➤ Alveolar pressure also affects capillary size.

Why are lung units with high V̇/Q̇ ratios unable to compensate for lung units with low V̇/Q̇ ratios?

When the pulmonary blood from lung units of varying V̇/Q̇ ratios mixes, the blood from areas of high V̇/Q̇ cannot compensate for the blood from areas of low V̇/Q̇ because it is the oxygen content of blood from the different areas that is mixed, not the partial pressures.

To illustrate this, imagine a hypothetical situation with two syringes of blood:

> Syringe A: 10 mL of blood with a PaO_2 of 5 kPa; oxygen content 15 mL
> Syringe B: 10 mL of blood with a PaO_2 of 15 kPa; oxygen content 20 mL

If we mix Syringes A and B the oxygen content of the resulting blood would be 17.5 mL, which would theoretically equate to a PaO_2 of approximately 8 kPa, i.e. PaO_2 is depressed below the mean value (which in this scenario should be 10 kPa).

With a patient in the lateral position, how is ventilation distributed in the following situations: awake patient, anaesthetised patient breathing spontaneously (GA/SV), anaesthetised and ventilated patient (GA/IPPV) and patient with an upper chest thoracotomy?

	Upper lung (V)	Lower lung (V)
Awake	40%	60%
GA/SV	55%	45%
GA/IPPV	60%	40%
Thoracotomy	70%	30%

Why are the above changes in ventilation distribution seen?

The explanation centres on the effect of anaesthesia on lung volume and hence the change in compliance of different areas of the lung. The lung pressure–volume curve illustrates the regional variation in lung compliance and shows how under anaesthesia the alveoli at the top of the lung (in the upper lung) move to a steeper portion of the compliance curve as their resting volume falls. Conversely, the basal alveoli (in the lower lung) move to a flatter, less compliant part of the curve.

Lung pressure–volume curve

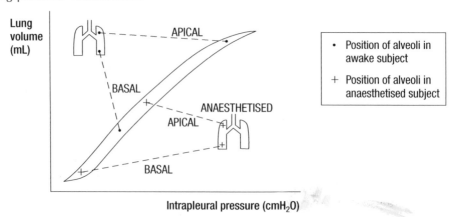

GRAPH 1.13 Lung pressure–volume curve illustrating the effect of anaesthesia on lung compliance

Note how under anaesthesia lung volume falls; the alveoli in the upper lung have a reduced volume resulting in increased compliance and hence improved ventilation. The alveoli in the lower lung also undergo volume reduction under anaesthesia. However, the reduction in volume leaves the lower lung alveoli less compliant and therefore ventilation is reduced.

What do you understand by the term 'shunt'?
Shunt is an extreme form of V̇/Q̇ mismatch, whereby blood enters the arterial system without passing through ventilated areas of the lung. It may be classified into intrapulmonary and extrapulmonary causes.

What are the causes of shunt?
Intrapulmonary:
➤ Physiological: Bronchial arterial blood passing into the pulmonary veins. Coronary venous blood draining into the left ventricle.
➤ Pathological: Lung collapse or consolidation with loss of ventilation.

Extrapulmonary:
➤ Cyanotic congenital heart disease, i.e. right to left intracardiac shunting, e.g. Tetralogy of Fallot.

What is the shunt equation?
The shunt equation allows the amount of shunt caused by the addition of venous blood to the arterial circulation to be calculated. It requires the subject to be breathing 100% oxygen. Of fundamental importance is the fact that of all of the causes of hypoxia, shunt cannot be corrected by breathing 100% oxygen because the shunted blood bypasses ventilated alveoli and thus is never exposed to the higher alveolar PO_2. The shunted blood therefore continues to depress the arterial oxygen content.

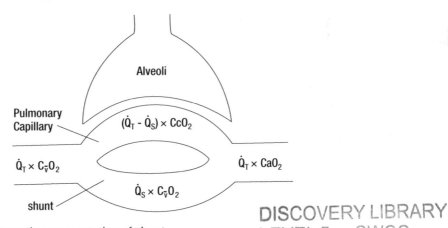

FIGURE 1.14 Schematic representation of shunt

$$\frac{\dot{Q}_S}{\dot{Q}_T} = \frac{CcO_2 - C_aO_2}{CcO_2 - C\bar{v}O_2}$$

Where:
$\dot{Q}_T$ Total blood flow (measured via cardiac output monitors)
$\dot{Q}_S$ Shunt blood flow
CcO_2 End-capillary oxygen content (estimated from alveolar gas eq.)
CaO_2 Arterial oxygen content (ABG then calculate oxygen content)

$C\bar{v}O_2$ – Mixed venous oxygen content (mixed venous blood sample from a PAFC then calculate venous oxygen content).

Can you draw the iso-shunt diagram?

The iso-shunt diagram demonstrates the arterial oxygen tension based on a given inspired oxygen fraction in the presence of various degrees of shunt:

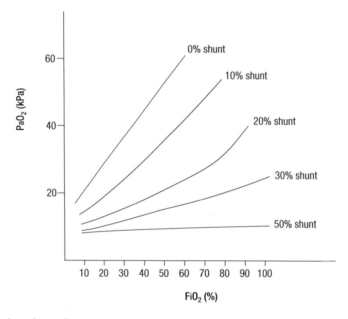

FIGURE 1.15 Iso-shunt diagram

CHAPTER 8

Respiratory dead space

Questions on respiratory dead space are particularly common in the primary FRCA examination. Examiners will expect clear definitions of what constitutes the different types of dead space and how they can be measured.

Define dead space as applied to the respiratory system

Respiratory dead space is the volume of inspired gas that takes no part in gas exchange. It is divided into anatomical and alveolar dead space.

➤ Anatomical dead space:
  ● constitutes the conducting airways (Weibel classification – airway generations 1–16: trachea; bronchi; bronchioles and terminal bronchioles)
  ● includes the mouth, nose and pharynx
  ● equates to 2 mL/kg.
➤ Anatomical dead space is increased by:
  ● sitting up
  ● neck extension
  ● jaw protrusion
  ● increasing age
  ● increasing lung volume.
➤ Anatomical dead space is decreased by:
  ● general anaesthesia
  ● hypoventilation
  ● intubation
  ● tracheostomy.
➤ Alveolar dead space:
  ● constitutes alveoli which are ventilated but not perfused and therefore no gas exchange occurs
  ● can be significantly affected by physiological and pathological processes.
➤ Physiological dead space:
  ● represents the combination of anatomical and alveolar dead space.

How is anatomical dead space measured?

Fowler's method is used to measure anatomical dead space. It is a technique which employs single breath nitrogen washout utilising a rapid nitrogen gas analyser.

➤ A nose clip is placed on the subject, and the subject breathes air in and out through their mouth via a mouthpiece.
➤ From the end of a normal expiratory breath (i.e. FRC) the subject takes a maximal breath of 100% O_2 to vital capacity.
➤ Subject then exhales maximally at a slow and constant rate to residual volume.
➤ During exhalation the expired gas passes through the rapid nitrogen analyser and so nitrogen concentration is measured against volume.
➤ Four distinct phases are seen in expired nitrogen concentration.

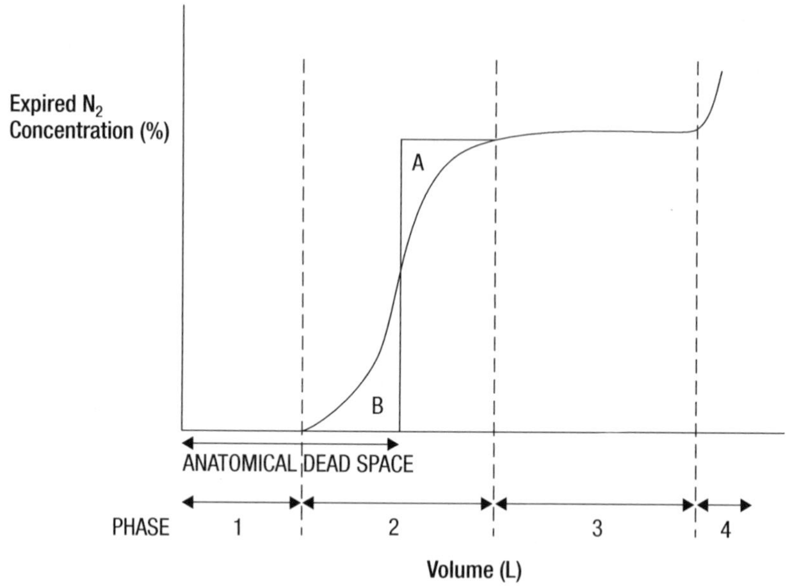

GRAPH 1.16 Nitrogen concentration versus lung volume

➤ **Phase 1:** Initial expired gas from the conducting airways containing 100% O_2 and no N_2.
➤ **Phase 2:** Nitrogen concentration increases as alveolar gas begins to mix with anatomical dead space gas.
➤ **Phase 3:** Alveolar plateau phase – exhalation of alveolar gas containing N_2 from the alveoli. Oscillations can be seen in phase 3 which are caused by interference from the heartbeat.
➤ **Phase 4:** Represents closing capacity. During expiration airways at the lung bases close as the lung approaches residual volume, so phase 4 expired gas comes mainly from the upper lung regions. During normal inspiration the lung bases are preferentially ventilated and therefore the lung apices receive less of the 100% O_2 breath. At closing volume N_2 from the lung apices is expired causing the phase 4 rise in expired N_2 concentration.
➤ **Anatomical dead space** is found by dividing phase 2 so that areas A and B are equal, and measuring from the start of exhalation.

How is physiological dead space measured?
The Bohr equation is used to derive physiological dead space (anatomical + alveolar).

$$\frac{V_{D.PHYS}}{V_T} = \frac{PaCO_2 - P_ECO_2}{PaCO_2}$$

Where:
$V_{D.PHYS}$ Physiological dead space
V_T Tidal volume – measured with a spirometer
$PaCO_2$ Arterial partial pressure of CO_2 – measured from an arterial blood gas
P_ECO_2 Mixed expired partial pressure of CO_2 – measured from end-tidal CO_2.

Any of the situations previously mentioned which increase anatomical dead space will consequently increase physiological dead space.

Alveolar dead space is increased by most lung diseases (especially pulmonary embolus), general anaesthesia, positive pressure ventilation and positive end expiratory pressure. Under such circumstances $V_{D.PHYS}/V_T$ may approach 70% (normally 35%), which has obvious implications for CO_2 removal.

CHAPTER 9

Lung volumes

Draw a spirometer trace to illustrate the various lung volumes
Spirometry is the standard method for measuring most relative lung volumes. However, it is incapable of providing information about absolute volumes of air in the lung. Thus a different approach is required to measure residual volume, functional residual capacity and total lung capacity. Two of the most common methods of obtaining information about these volumes are gas dilution tests and body plethysmography.

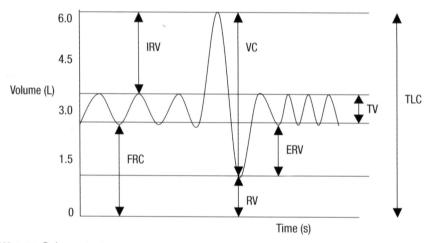

GRAPH 1.17 Spirometry trace

All values quoted are approximate for a 70 kg male:
TLC   Total lung capacity (6000 mL)
VC   Vital capacity (4800 mL)
TV   Tidal volume (400–600 mL)
IRV   Inspiratory reserve volume (2500 mL)
ERV   Expiratory reserve volume (1200 mL)
RV   Residual volume (1200–1500 mL)
FRC   Functional residual capacity (3000 mL standing up/2000 mL supine).

Which lung volumes can be measured with a spirometer?
Any lung volume which incorporates residual volume cannot be measured with simple spirometry (i.e. TLC, RV and FRC), the rest can be measured:
➤ **vital capacity** – the maximum volume expired after a maximal inspiration
➤ **tidal volume** – normal resting breath volume
➤ **inspiratory reserve volume** – volume of air that can be inspired over and above the resting tidal volume
➤ **expiratory reserve volume** – volume of air that can be expired from FRC.

How can absolute lung volumes be measured?

The absolute lung volumes are:

➤ **residual volume** – volume of air remaining in the lungs after maximal expiration

➤ **total lung capacity** – total volume of air in the lungs after maximal inspiration

➤ **functional residual capacity** – volume of air remaining in the lungs after a normal expiratory breath.

They cannot be measured by simple spirometry, but require the use of more advanced techniques such as **gas dilution** or **body plethysmography**.

Describe how nitrogen washout may be used to measure RV and FRC

➤ The fractional lung nitrogen concentration (FLN$_2$) is constant at 79% (i.e. 790 mL per 1000 mL air). The subject rebreathes several times from a bag of known volume containing a nitrogen-free gas. Thus, the nitrogen from the patient's lungs equilibrates with gas in the bag and so the nitrogen concentration will decrease as the volume of distribution has increased.

➤ In order to measure RV, the rebreathing process is started from the end of a maximal expiration (i.e. from RV).

➤ In order to measure FRC, the rebreathing process is started from the end of a normal tidal breath (i.e. from FRC).

➤ The principle behind the nitrogen washout method is that the amount of nitrogen at the start of the determination (nitrogen in the patient's lungs only) is the same amount that ultimately is distributed between the lung and the bag. As the volume of the bag and the fractional concentration of nitrogen in the lungs are known, the fractional concentration of nitrogen in the bag at equilibration is measured, allowing calculation of either RV or FRC.

Thus:

$$VL = \frac{VB \times FxN_2}{FLN_2 - FxN_2}$$

Where:

VL   Volume of lung (FRC or RV)
VB   Volume of bag
FxN$_2$ Fractional concentration of N$_2$ in bag
FLN$_2$ Fractional concentration of N$_2$ in the lung.

Exactly the same principle is utilised for the **helium wash-in method** of determining RV or FRC. Both the nitrogen washout and helium wash-in methods only measure communicating gas. This is a disadvantage compared to the total body plethysmography method, which is able to measure communicating and non-communicating gas (i.e. gas trapped behind closed airways).

In body plethysmography

➤ The subject sits inside an airtight chamber equipped to measure pressure, flow, or volume changes.

➤ The subject inhales or exhales to a particular volume (usually FRC), and then a shutter drops across their breathing tube.

➤ The subject makes respiratory efforts against the closed shutter, causing their chest volume to expand and decompressing the air in their lungs.

➤ The increase in their chest volume slightly reduces the box volume and thus slightly increases the pressure in the box.
➤ The most common measurements made using the body plethysmograph are thoracic gas volume (VTG) and airway resistance (Raw).

The following equation is then used:

$$\text{Pressure } 1 \times \text{Volume } 1 = \text{Pressure } 2 \times (\text{Volume } 1 - \text{Volume } 2)$$

(It utilises Boyle's Law – at a constant temperature, within a closed system, pressure is inversely proportional to volume.)

What determines FRC?
FRC is dependent on the balance of the tendency of the lungs to recoil and the thoracic cage to expand.

Under conditions of apnoea, FRC represents the pulmonary oxygen store. If FRC is 2500 mL, breathing 21% O_2 the oxygen store is 500 mL, but this can be increased by pre-oxygenation (denitrogenation) to 2500 mL. If resting total body O_2 requirement is 250 mL/min, FRC represents a 10 minute O_2 store during apnoea.

FRC is increased by:
➤ standing position
➤ COPD
➤ asthma
➤ PEEP.

FRC is reduced by:
➤ supine position
➤ general anaesthesia
➤ pregnancy
➤ obesity.

What is closing capacity?
The closing capacity is the volume of the lungs at which the small airways begin to collapse and close off. If FRC is less than the closing capacity, areas of the lung will be perfused but not ventilated, resulting in an increase in $\dot{V}/\dot{Q}$ mismatch.

CHAPTER 10

Lung compliance

Define compliance as applied to the respiratory system

Compliance is defined as the change in volume per unit change in transpulmonary pressure. Units mL/cmH$_2$O. Normal lung compliance is 200 mL/cmH$_2$O.

➤ **Specific compliance** is compliance divided by FRC, thereby compensating for differing body sizes.
➤ **Elastance** is the reciprocal of compliance.

The most important determinant of lung compliance is the surface tension of the alveolar fluid. Lung surfactant greatly reduces surface tension at the air–tissue interface and thus increases lung compliance. The effects of lack of pulmonary surfactant are clearly evident in conditions such as neonatal respiratory distress syndrome.

Draw a pressure–volume curve of the lung

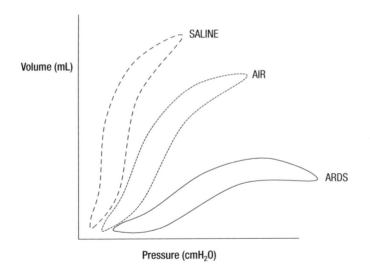

GRAPH 1.18 Lung pressure–volume curves

➤ The slope of the pressure–volume curve equates to lung compliance.
➤ Note how in ARDS lung compliance is greatly reduced; conversely in hypothetical saline filled lungs, compliance is greatly increased.

What do you understand by the term hysteresis?

At any given lung volume, the pressure required to inflate the lung is greater than the pressure required for deflation.

What is the difference between static and dynamic compliance?
➤ **Static compliance** is measured when all gas flow in the lungs has ceased.
➤ **Dynamic compliance** is measured when gas flow at the mouth is zero (at end-expiration or end-inspiration) but during rhythmic respiration.
➤ Static compliance is always greater than dynamic compliance and the reason for this is the variation of time constants in different areas of the lung.
➤ Dynamic compliance falls as respiratory rate increases, mainly because of tissue resistance (i.e. mechanical properties of lung tissue are time-dependent) and differing time constants of different areas of lung.

$$\text{Time constant} = \text{Resistance} \times \text{Compliance}$$

How can static and dynamic compliance be measured?
➤ **Static compliance:** Intrapleural pressure can be estimated from oesophageal pressure (oesophageal pressure probe). The subject then breathes out from total lung capacity into a spirometer, thus pressure and volume are measured and subsequently plotted to produce a pressure–volume curve from which compliance is determined.
➤ **Dynamic compliance:** During rhythmic breathing, again intrapleural pressure is estimated from oesophageal pressure. However, now the pressure is measured at no-flow points (end-inspiration or end-expiration). At these points in the respiratory cycle, intrapleural pressure reflects lung elastic recoil forces. The volume difference divided by pressure difference at these points equates to compliance.

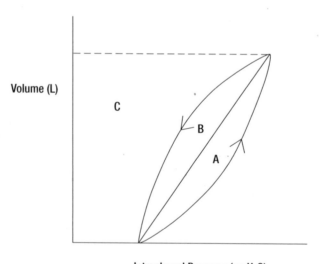

Volume (L)

C

B

A

Intrapleural Pressure (cmH$_2$0)

GRAPH 1.19 Lung pressure–volume curve

➤ **Work of breathing:** The work of breathing is defined by the area to the left of the pressure–volume curve. The normal metabolic cost of breathing is approximately 0.5–1.0 mL O$_2$/L/min but this may increase to 2–4 mL O$_2$/L/min with hyperventilation.
➤ **Inspiration:** Work required to overcome the elastic recoil of the chest wall and lungs; airways resistance (areas A and C).
➤ **Expiration:** Passive under resting conditions (area B). Active during stress conditions.
➤ Work increases with increasing tidal volume, and with increasing respiratory flow.

CHAPTER 11

Control of respiration

• Describe the control of respiration
This is a straightforward question so keep it simple!
  ➤ Ventilation is regulated in order to maintain homeostasis of pH, PaO_2 and $PaCO_2$ in the blood.
  ➤ The respiratory centre is located in the brainstem and is composed of a group of nuclei within the medulla and pons.
  ➤ Three major brainstem respiratory neuronal areas have been identified:
    • **dorsal respiratory group (DRG) of neurons** – located in the medulla and controls inspiration
    • **pneumotaxic area** – located in the pons and assists in regulating inspiration
    • **ventral respiratory group (VRG) of neurons** – located in the medulla and regulates expiration.
  ➤ The respiratory centre receives input from peripheral and central chemoreceptors.

Brainstem
  ➤ Medulla – DRG of neurons controls inspiration. This area has intrinsic automaticity and exhibits a ramp effect of increasing action potential frequency to the diaphragm and other inspiratory muscles and is responsible for basic ventilatory rhythm.
  ➤ Inspiration may be terminated prematurely by inhibiting impulses from the pneumotaxic centre. In effect, the pneumotaxic centre 'fine tunes' inspiration.
  ➤ During normal quiet breathing expiration is passive. However, during exercise, for example, the VRG of neurones become active and expiratory muscles are stimulated.

Peripheral chemoreceptors
  ➤ Located in the aortic (near aortic arch) and carotid bodies (bifurcation of the common carotid). Cranial nerves X and IX respectively link the receptors to the brainstem.
  ➤ The peripheral chemoreceptors primarily respond to hypoxia and respond to partial pressure of oxygen in the arterial blood rather than oxygen content of the blood. Thus patients suffering from reduced blood oxygen content due to anaemia or carboxyhaemoglobin do not have respiratory stimulation via the peripheral chemoreceptors.
  ➤ The chemoreceptors are composed of glomus cells, which contain dopamine.
  ➤ Each carotid body receives an extremely high blood flow equivalent to $2\,L/100\,g$ tissue/ minute.
  ➤ The aortic bodies respond to reductions in PaO_2 and rises in $PaCO_2$ by stimulating the inspiratory centre to increase respiratory rate.
  ➤ The carotid bodies respond not only to reductions in PaO_2 and rises in $PaCO_2$, but also to pH changes.
  ➤ Hypotension may also result in stimulation of the peripheral chemoreceptors probably via stagnant hypoxia.

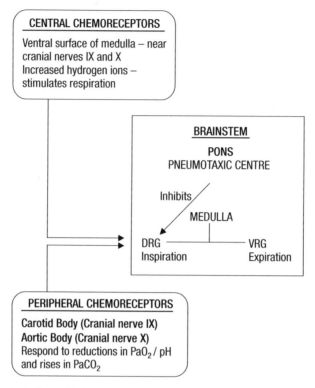

FIGURE 1.20 Control of respiration

➤ The respiratory stimulant doxapram acts via the peripheral chemoreceptors.
➤ Volatile anaesthetics abolish the peripheral chemoreceptor response to hypoxia.

Central chemoreceptors
➤ Situated in the ventral medulla, in an area that is extremely sensitive to hydrogen ions.
➤ Chemoreceptors are surrounded by extracellular fluid.
➤ When blood $PaCO_2$ rises, CO_2 diffuses across the blood brain barrier into the CSF generating hydrogen ions [$CO_2 + H_2O \leftrightharpoons H_2CO_3 \leftrightharpoons H + HCO_3$].
➤ pH thus falls (note that CSF has less protein than blood and therefore less buffering capacity) and this stimulates the inspiratory area.
➤ Hypercarbia provides an acute drive to increase ventilation for up to 48 hours; after this period CSF compensation occurs via increased HCO_3 transport into the CSF in order to correct pH.

Voluntary control of respiration
➤ Cerebral cortex can override brainstem control, within limits, e.g. voluntary hyperventilation.
➤ Limbic system and hypothalamus – emotions such as rage and fear may also alter respiratory pattern.

Describe the response to inhalation of 5% CO_2 in oxygen

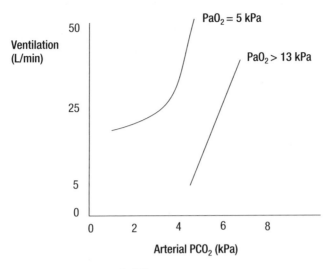

GRAPH 1.21 Ventilatory response to $PaCO_2$

➤ Over a short period of time, $PaCO_2$ will increase, which in turn will lead to an increase in CSF hydrogen ion concentration and thus a fall in pH which will be detected by the central chemoreceptors, leading to an increase in respiratory rate.

➤ An additional stimulus to respiration will come from the peripheral chemoreceptors, which will detect both the rise in $PaCO_2$ and the fall in pH, leading to input to the DRG of neurons via cranial nerves IX and X.

➤ Note that the ventilatory response to CO_2 is reduced by opiates, increasing age and sleep.

Describe the effects of raised CO_2 on the body
➤ Hypercarbia stimulates respiration via activation of peripheral and central chemoreceptors.
➤ CVS – Systemic vasodilatation, myocardial depression and arrhythmias.
➤ Pulmonary circulation – Increased pulmonary vascular resistance.
➤ Respiratory acidosis.
➤ CNS – Stimulates respiration but at high levels causes narcosis. Increases cerebral blood flow and intracranial pressure.
➤ Renal – Slower compensation via bicarbonate retention and urinary hydrogen ion excretion.

Describe the ventilatory response to hypoxia
➤ Hypoxaemia stimulates ventilation through its effects on the carotid and aortic bodies (peripheral chemoreceptors). Hypoxaemia is not a stimulus for the central chemoreceptors, although prolonged hypoxia will cause cerebral acidosis, which in turn can stimulate respiration.
➤ Isocapnic (holding CO_2 constant) oxygen curves illustrate the effect of changing PaO_2 on alveolar ventilation. The main stimulation of respiration through hypoxia occurs at $PaO_2 < 8\,kPa$. Hypercarbia augments the ventilatory response to hypoxia.

➤ Increasing $PaCO_2$ by 0.1 kPa results in an increase in alveolar ventilation of approximately 1–2 L/min. In the same way a reduction in $PaCO_2$ results in a reduction in alveolar ventilation up until a $PaCO_2$ of 4 kPa below which there is no effect. Hypoxia produces a higher alveolar ventilation for any given $PaCO_2$.

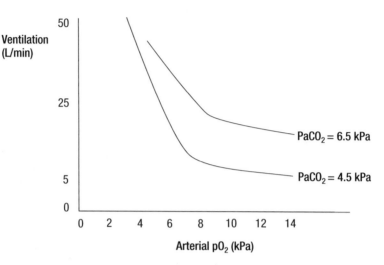

GRAPH 1.22 Ventilatory response to PaO_2

CHAPTER 12

Altitude and diving

Two extremes! The application of respiratory physiology principles to these two unusual environments requires a good understanding of the basic concepts of respiratory physiology and therefore is a popular examination question.

Altitude
The highest permanent habitation in the world is found in the Andes Mountain Range at 4877 m (16 000 ft) above sea level. In the northern Andes, the majority of inhabitants live above 2743 m (9000 ft). The capital cities of Bolivia (La Paz), Ecuador (Quito) and Colombia (Bogotá) are all high altitude cities. La Paz is the highest capital city in the world at 3630 m (11 910 ft).

➤ Atmospheric pressure halves every 5500 m (18 000 ft).
➤ The percentage of oxygen in the atmosphere at sea level is about 21% and the barometric pressure is around 101 kPa. As altitude increases, the percentage remains the same but the number of oxygen molecules per breath is reduced. At 3600 m (12 000 ft) the barometric pressure is only about 64 kPa (480 mmHg), so there are roughly 40% fewer oxygen molecules per breath thus the body must adjust to having less oxygen.
➤ At 19 200 m (63 000 ft) barometric pressure is 6.25 kPa, meaning inspired PiO₂ is zero.

If a human being who resides at sea level were to be suddenly dropped on to the top of Mount Everest (8848 m/29 028 ft) he or she would succumb to hypoxia and lose consciousness. The body requires a period of acclimatisation during which physiological adaptation occurs in response to the relative lack of oxygen.

Describe the acute and chronic physiological responses to high altitude
The alveolar gas equation is key to understanding the fundamental physiological response to high altitude:

$$P_AO_2 = PiO_2 - \frac{P_ACO_2}{R}$$

Where:
P_AO_2 Alveolar partial pressure of oxygen
PiO_2 Inspired pressure of oxygen = $FiO_2 \times (P_{ATM} - P_{H2O})$ fraction of inspired oxygen multiplied by the difference between atmospheric pressure and water vapour pressure
P_ACO_2 Alveolar partial pressure of carbon dioxide (approximates with arterial CO_2)
R Respiratory Quotient = CO_2 production / O_2 consumption (N=0.8).

➤ **Hyperventilation:** On ascent to altitude there is an increase in minute ventilation as a result of hypoxic stimulation of the peripheral chemoreceptors located in the aortic and carotid bodies. The hyperventilation results in a lowered arterial $PaCO_2$, which increases alveolar pressure of oxygen, as can be seen from the alveolar gas equation. The hypocarbia secondary to hyperventilation results in CSF alkalosis. However, this is transient as bicarbonate is excreted from the CSF over 24–48 hours and renally excreted.

➤ **Oxyhaemoglobin dissociation curve:** At moderate altitudes there is a right shift in the oxyhaemoglobin dissociation curve caused by increased levels of 2,3 DPG, thereby favouring oxygen unloading.

At high altitudes there is an overall left shift in the oxyhaemoglobin dissociation curve favouring oxygen uptake in the pulmonary capillaries.

➤ **Polycythaemia:** Increased erythropoietin secretion results in a slow increase in red cell count in order to increase oxygen-carrying capacity. However, this also results in a raised haematocrit, which can lead to thrombosis.

➤ **Cardiovascular responses:** Increase in heart rate and stroke volume from sympathetic stimulation from the effects of hypoxia in an attempt to maintain oxygen delivery to the tissues. Overall rise in myocardial work.

➤ **Hypoxic pulmonary vasoconstriction:** Results in an increase in pulmonary vascular resistance, which can lead to right heart failure.

➤ **Angiogenesis and enzyme changes:** Increase in capillary density with time thereby reducing oxygen diffusion distance. This is associated with a change in intracellular oxidative enzymes favouring cellular respiration under hypoxic conditions.

How does high altitude affect volatile anaesthesia?

➤ Gas and vapour analysers measure partial pressure and assume sea level atmospheric pressure (101 kPa). E.g. an oxygen analyser measuring 21 kPa will assume atmospheric pressure to be 101 kPa and provide a percentage of oxygen on the display of 21% or 0.21. However, if the analyser is used at an altitude where atmospheric pressure is only 70 kPa, the analyser will under-read, displaying 21% when it should be 33%.

➤ TEC vaporisers function normally at altitude. The output of these vaporisers is a constant partial pressure of volatile agent *not* a constant volume percentage.

E.g. Vaporiser dialled to deliver 1% isoflurane:

• gas from the vaporising chamber is fully saturated with volatile agent (i.e. it has achieved its saturated vapour pressure (SVP) at that ambient temperature)
• SVP is not affected by ambient pressure (i.e. does not change with altitude)
• 1% isoflurane at sea level will have a partial pressure of 1%
• 1% isoflurane at altitude – the volatile agent from the vaporising chamber will be diluted into a less dense gas stream and therefore the concentration of isoflurane will be higher but the partial pressure remains the same as it would be at sea level. Clinical effect is dependent on the partial pressure and therefore remains the same.

What is acute mountain sickness (AMS)?

AMS is very common at high altitude. At over 3000 m (10 000 ft) 75% of people will have mild symptoms. The occurrence of AMS is dependent upon the elevation, the rate of ascent and individual susceptibility. Many people will experience mild AMS during the acclimatisation process. The symptoms usually start 12 to 24 hours after arrival at altitude and begin to decrease in severity around the third day. The symptoms of mild AMS include:

➤ headache
➤ nausea and dizziness
➤ loss of appetite
➤ fatigue
➤ shortness of breath
➤ disturbed sleep
➤ general feeling of malaise.

What is high altitude pulmonary oedema (HAPO)?

HAPO results from increased pulmonary extravascular lung water, which prevents effective oxygen exchange. As the condition progresses, severe hypoxaemia develops which leads to cyanosis, impaired cerebral function and death. Symptoms of HAPO include:

➤ shortness of breath at rest
➤ tightness in the chest and a persistent cough bringing up white, watery or frothy fluid
➤ marked fatigue and weakness
➤ a feeling of impending suffocation at night
➤ confusion and irrational behaviour.

What is high altitude cerebral oedema (HACO)?

HACO is a potentially life-threatening complication of high altitude resulting from swelling of brain tissue secondary to fluid leakage. Symptoms of HACO include:

➤ headache
➤ weakness
➤ disorientation
➤ loss of coordination
➤ decreasing levels of consciousness
➤ loss of memory
➤ hallucinations and psychotic behaviour
➤ coma.

Describe the treatment of AMS

The only cure for mountain sickness is either acclimatisation or descent. Symptoms of mild AMS can be treated with analgesics for headache (e.g. ibuprofen), acetazolamide and dexamethasone.

➤ **Acetazolamide:** carbonic anhydrase inhibitor, which reduces bicarbonate formation and increases hydrogen ion concentration in the body leading to development of a metabolic acidosis, which causes a respiratory compensation response resulting in an increase in minute ventilation and thus further lowering of $PaCO_2$.
➤ **Dexamethasone:** corticosteroid with predominantly glucocorticoid actions. It has anti-inflammatory properties and is useful in reducing cerebral oedema. Many pilgrims at the annual festival at Gosainkunda lake in Nepal suffer from HACO following a rapid rate of ascent, and respond remarkably well to dexamethasone.

Other treatments for altitude sickness include the following

➤ **Nifedipine:** calcium channel blocker, most commonly used as an anti-hypertensive. It also has the effect of rapidly reducing pulmonary artery pressure by inhibiting hypoxic pulmonary vasoconstriction, thereby improving oxygen transfer. It can therefore be used to treat HAPO, though unfortunately its effectiveness is not anywhere as dramatic as that of dexamethasone in HACO.
➤ **Furosemide:** loop diuretic, may be used to treat pulmonary oedema acutely. However, furosemide may also lead to collapse from low volume shock if the victim is already dehydrated.
➤ **100% oxygen** also reduces the effects of altitude sickness.

Diving

During diving the opposite problems to altitude are seen. Barometric pressure increases by 1 atmosphere for every 10 m of descent (e.g. at a depth of 30 m barometric pressure will be 4 atmospheres).

The following specific issues relate to respiratory physiology during diving:
➤ effects of compression and decompression
➤ inert gas narcosis
➤ decompression sickness
➤ oxygen toxicity
➤ high pressure nervous syndrome.

What mechanics are involved during compression and decompression?
During diving, as depth increases so too does barometric pressure. This increase in pressure is not a problem as long as it is balanced, i.e. there is no pressure gradient. Compression of gas-filled cavities such as the lungs, middle ear and sinuses will occur on descent. On rapid ascent the pressure difference between these cavities and barometric pressure may not have time to equilibrate, potentially resulting in complications such as pneumothoraces or perforated tympanic membranes.

What are the problems for scuba divers using an air mixture at depth?
Air contains 79% nitrogen. At high barometric pressures nitrogen has narcotic properties. This means that air can only be safely used up to a depth of 30–50 m.
At depths exceeding 50 m helium/oxygen gas mixtures are used. Helium does not exhibit the narcotic properties of nitrogen.

What limits the depth under water that a human can breathe via a snorkel?
A snorkel has an apparatus dead space, which means that if it is beyond a certain length, rebreathing of expired gas will occur, resulting in hypercarbia from impaired CO_2 elimination.

As the diver descends deeper under water, barometric pressure increases which increases pressure within the circulation. However, because the diver's lungs are exposed to atmospheric pressure via the snorkel, a situation develops whereby pulmonary vascular pressure is greater than alveolar pressure, causing pulmonary oedema.

It becomes difficult to breathe via a snorkel at depths exceeding 1 m as a result of the compression·effects on the chest.

Describe the physiology of decompression sickness
➤ At depths exceeding 20 m nitrogen is absorbed into body tissues, especially fat. However, nitrogen has a low solubility and therefore equilibration between environment and body takes hours. If rapid ascent occurs, nitrogen comes out of solution forming bubbles. These bubbles can cause severe microvascular complications by obstructing blood flow; in the brain this can lead to visual disturbances or convulsions; joint pain can be severe.
➤ Treatment of decompression sickness is recompression, which forces nitrogen back into solution.
➤ Using a non-air gas mixture such as helium-oxygen reduces the risk of decompression sickness. Helium is 50% less soluble than nitrogen so less is dissolved into tissues, reducing subsequent risk.
➤ As a rough rule of thumb it is safe for a diver to rapidly halve their ambient pressure, e.g. a rapid ascent from 10 m depth (2 atm) to the surface (1 atm).
➤ Commercial saturation divers who work at great depths live in high-pressure chambers so that their bodies remain saturated in nitrogen, thus avoiding decompression sickness. At the end of their period of diving they decompress, a process which will take a considerable amount of time!

What would happen if a diver performing a breath hold dive hyperventilated prior to the dive?

Competitive apnoea is an extreme sport in which competitors attempt to attain great depths, times or distances on a single breath without direct assistance of self-contained underwater breathing apparatus (scuba).

The adaptations made by the human body while under water and at high pressure include:

➤ bradycardia
➤ vasoconstriction: redistribution of blood flow to myocardium, lungs and brain
➤ splenic contraction.

The record breath hold dive is 140 m. Hyperventilating prior to such a dive is not a sensible manoeuvre! Hyperventilation results in hypocarbia. The normal stimulus to terminate descent and commence ascent would be the development of hypoxia and hypercarbia. If the diver hyperventilated prior to such a dive the only stimulus to ascend would be hypoxia. On ascent as barometric pressure falls so too would alveolar inspired oxygen (via alveolar gas equation), resulting in severe hypoxaemia and possible hypoxic seizures on ascent or even loss of consciousness.

Can oxygen toxicity develop during diving?

Yes.

➤ At oxygen partial pressure of greater than 2 atmospheres oxygen toxicity is a risk; this equates to air diving at depths greater than 40 m (=5 atm / PO_2 > 2 atm). CNS excitation can lead to nausea, tinnitus, twitching and convulsions.
➤ The exact aetiology of the CNS toxicity from hyperoxia is not fully understood.

The implication for divers is the use of a hypoxic gas mixture to overcome this problem. For increasingly deep dives the oxygen concentration in the tank will be less than 21% and at extreme depths as low as 1%!

What is the physiological basis for hyperbaric oxygen therapy?

Increasing the arterial partial pressure of oxygen via increasing barometric pressure has a number of effects:

➤ increases amount of dissolved oxygen
➤ improves oxygen diffusion (Fick's Law of Diffusion)
➤ promotes angiogenesis
➤ improves function of polymorphs
➤ inhibits growth of anaerobes (useful in gas gangrene)
➤ displaces carbon monoxide from haemoglobin.

At a barometric pressure of 3 atm there is sufficient dissolved oxygen alone to meet body oxygen requirements. May be of use in a Jehovah's Witness patient with an acute perioperative anaemia refusing blood transfusion.

What are some of the clinical indications for hyperbaric oxygen therapy?
➤ **Gas lesions:** air or gas emboli; decompression sickness.
➤ **Infections:** refractory osteomyelitis; necrotising soft tissue infections; clostridial infections.
➤ **Global hypoxia:** carbon monoxide poisoning; severe anaemia.
➤ **Regional hypoxia:** compromised grafts or free flaps; osteoradionecrosis; crush injuries.

What are the contraindications to hyperbaric oxygen therapy?
➤ untreated pneumothorax
➤ gas trapping in the lungs, e.g. lung bullae/bronchospasm
➤ unusual drugs, e.g. doxorubicin.

CHAPTER 13

Lung function measurement

How would you assess and measure a patient's lung function?
The aim of pre-operative lung function testing is to identify patients at high risk of periop-erative pulmonary complications, in order to attempt to reduce perioperative risk via good patient preparation pre-operatively, targeted anaesthetic and surgical techniques intraopera-tively, and planning for the required level of care post-operatively (e.g. HDU/ITU). If patient risk is high and the risk cannot be reduced, the risk–benefit ratio for surgery needs to be carefully evaluated and a decision made as to whether to proceed.

Evaluation of a patient's pulmonary function requires correlation of history, examination findings and relevant investigation results.

Clinical
History and examination findings may provide valuable information about a patient's res-piratory function. Pertinent history should include history of pre-existing lung disease (e.g. COPD, asthma, pulmonary fibrosis), smoking history (quantified via pack-year history), exercise tolerance, respiratory symptoms (cough, sputum production, wheeze), number and frequency of hospital admissions with respiratory problems, and current treatment regimen (e.g. bronchodilators, steroids, supplemental oxygen etc.)

Risk factors for pulmonary complications include the following
Patient factors:
➤ age > 70 years
➤ history of lung disease
➤ BMI > 30
➤ smoking history > 20-pack year.

Surgical factors:
➤ upper abdominal surgery
➤ thoracic surgery
➤ open vs. laparoscopic procedures.

Investigations
Investigations should be targeted to the patient, i.e. based on clinical assessment and based upon the nature of the planned surgery. Investigations, which will have little or no clinical impact, should be avoided. For example, a CXR in a 20-year-old ASA 1 patient presenting for femoral hernia repair would be inappropriate. However, a CXR may well be indicated in a 20-year-old patient with cystic fibrosis presenting for the same procedure.

Peak expiratory flow rate (PEFR)
PEFR provides a simple method to measure airways obstruction, particularly in asthmatic patients. Normal range values are dependent on age, sex and height. It is particularly useful in asthmatic patients.

20-year-old female height 1.60 m PEFR 433 L/min
20-year-old male height 1.83 m PEFR 654 L/min

Arterial blood gas (ABG) analysis

Allows evaluation of gas exchange by providing essential information about the state of oxygenation, acid–base balance and severity of respiratory failure. It is extremely useful to have baseline arterial blood gases, especially for patients undergoing surgery, where there will inevitably be perioperative changes in gas exchange, the baseline arterial gases allowing easier interpretation of any subsequent changes.

Spirometry

➤ Spirometry is the timed measurement of dynamic lung volumes during forced expiration and inspiration.
➤ Measurements – forced vital capacity (FVC), forced expiratory volume in one second (FEV1) and the ratio of these two volumes (FEV1/FVC).
➤ Measurement of maximum expiratory flow over the middle 50% of the vital capacity (FEF25–75%) is a sensitive index of small airway function.
➤ Measures of forced maximal flow during expiration and inspiration flow can be made as a function of volume thus generating a flow volume curve, the shape of which also contains information of diagnostic value (*see* 'Interpretation of spirometry data').

Interpretation of spirometry data

➤ The presence of ventilatory abnormality can be implied if any of FEV1, FVC, or FEV1/VC ratio are outside the reference ranges.
➤ Interrelationships of the various measurements are important diagnostically:
  • FEV1/FVC < 80% constitutes an obstructive ventilatory defect (e.g. asthma/COPD)
  • FEV1/FVC > 80% constitutes a restrictive ventilatory defect (e.g. pulmonary fibrosis/kyphoscoliosis).

It is routine practice to quantify the degree of reversibility of an obstructive defect by measuring spirometry before and after the administration of a bronchodilator.

Generally, an improvement in FEV1 of 200 mL or more infers significant reversibility if the baseline FEV1 is < 1.5 L, as does an improvement of > 15% if the FEV1 is > 1.5 L.

Flow volume loops

Flow volume loops are constructed from spirometric data. Note that expiratory flow is above the x-axis, whereas inspiratory flow is represented below the x-axis. Analysis of the flow volume loops can be diagnostic.

Cardiopulmonary exercise testing (CPET)

Cardiopulmonary exercise testing is a non-invasive and objective method of evaluating both cardiac and pulmonary function. In practice, CPET testing should be considered when specific questions remain unanswered after consideration of basic clinical data. Cycle ergometry is the most common mode of exercise. CPET is a safe procedure, with the risk of death for patients between 2 and 5 per 100 000 exercise tests performed. This computerised test provides a breath-by-breath analysis of respiratory gas exchange at rest and during a period of exercise, the intensity of which is increased incrementally until symptoms limit testing or the patient reaches maximal levels. Information on airflow, O_2 consumption, CO_2 production, and heart rate are collected and used for computation of other variables such as oxygen uptake and the anaerobic threshold. CPET primarily determines if the patient has normal or reduced maximal exercise capacity ($\dot{V}O_2$ max). Reduced $\dot{V}O_2$ max can further suggest probable causes. CPET is used to define which organ systems (pulmonary or cardiac) contribute to a patient's symptoms of exertional dyspnea and exercise intolerance and to what extent. The anaerobic threshold may also be measured using CPET. The test is also

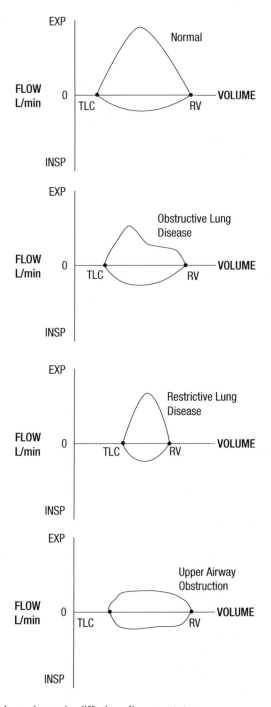

GRAPH 1.23 Flow volume loops in differing disease states

more sensitive for detecting early or subclinical disease than are less comprehensive tests that are done at rest. CPET is establishing a key role in pre-operative assessment of high-risk patients undergoing major surgery.

Respiratory muscle strength

Respiratory muscle strength may be assessed globally by measurement of maximum mouth pressures. Maximum inspiratory mouth pressure measurements reflect the force-generating capacity of inspiratory muscles. Measurements are taken during maximum inspiratory effort against an occlusion at residual volume (where mechanical advantage of inspiratory muscles is greatest) or at FRC.

Carbon monoxide diffusing capacity (transfer factor)

The diffusing capacity for carbon monoxide (DLco) is a measure of the ability of gas to transfer from alveoli to red blood cells across the alveolar epithelium and the capillary endothelium.

The DLco depends not only on the area and thickness of the blood–gas barrier but also on the volume of blood in the pulmonary capillaries. The distribution of alveolar volume and ventilation also affects the measurement.

DLco is measured by sampling end-expiratory gas for carbon monoxide (CO) after a patient inspires a small amount of CO, holds their breath, and exhales. Measured DLco should be adjusted for alveolar volume (which is estimated from dilution of helium) and the patient's haematocrit. DLco is reported as mL/min/mmHg and as a percentage of a predicted value.

Conditions which are associated with a reduced DLco

➤ Primary pulmonary hypertension
➤ Pulmonary embolism
➤ Emphysema
➤ Pulmonary fibrosis

Conditions which are associated with an increased DLco

➤ Polycythaemia
➤ Alveolar haemorrhage

Within the perioperative context of lung function assessment, it should be remembered that the input of a respiratory physician might be invaluable.

CHAPTER 14

Effects of anaesthesia on lung function

Can you describe the effects of general anaesthesia on lung function?

General anaesthesia has multiple important effects on lung function. The easiest way to think of the changes is to divide them into categories:

Respiratory control

➤ The patient's basal metabolic rate drops by 15% following induction of anaesthesia, due to thalamic inhibition.
➤ The response to hypercapnia is blunted and the acute responses to acidosis and hypoxia are almost entirely abolished.

Lung mechanics

➤ Following induction, functional residual capacity (FRC) falls by 15–20% because there is a loss of muscle tone. This decreased tone reduces the bucket handle action of the rib cage, which consequently moves less; breathing is more dependent on the movement of the diaphragm, which is similarly weakened. Phasic activity develops in the expiratory muscles, which are normally silent.
➤ In spontaneous, awake ventilation, expiration is a passive movement; under anaesthesia it becomes an active one.
➤ Lung compliance is reduced and airway resistance increases slightly; these combine to increase the work of breathing.
➤ Muco-ciliary transport mechanisms are reduced, which can cause retention of secretions.

Gas exchange

➤ The changes described above can cause atelectasis, and inhibit hypoxic pulmonary vasoconstriction. Logically, the application of PEEP should improve the situation as it helps to 'splint' the alveoli open. However, applying PEEP will also reduce blood flow to the splinted areas, by altering the pressure across the alveoli and therefore capillary walls (remember Starling's resistors and West's Zones of the Lung). So PEEP may actually increase $\dot{V}/\dot{Q}$ mismatching and should be applied with care in unstable patients. As with all things, this is a balance of risk. The application of PEEP may also destabilise the cardiovascular system in a particularly sick patient. Without the application of any PEEP, around 10% of pulmonary blood is shunted or perfuses areas with low $\dot{V}/\dot{Q}$.
➤ Alveolar dead space rises from 0 to 70 mL and physiological dead space from 150 to 220 mL. Intubation decreases dead space, but this effect is reduced by connectors etc.

All the changes described are exaggerated in those patients with lung disease.

Smokers should be counselled to stop smoking at least 6 weeks prior to their operations to allow their muco-ciliary and inflammatory cell function to return to somewhere approaching normal. Failing this, they should definitely not smoke for at least 12 hours prior to surgery, as the half-life of carbon monoxide is 4 hours.

In all patients, the effects of anaesthesia on lung function will last a few hours post-operatively. After major surgery, or in those with lung disease, the effects may last many days.

If the patient is placed on their side on the table, how will their position affect the flow of gases into the lungs?

➤ The flow of gases is dependent upon whether the patient is spontaneously breathing or being ventilated with positive pressure.

➤ If the patient is spontaneously ventilating, gas will be drawn into the dependent lung, i.e. the lowermost lung. The situation is reversed, however, when the patient is ventilated. Now gas will follow the path of least resistance into the non-dependent lung, whose total compliance would be greater as it does not have the weight of the thorax pressing down on it. As blood is preferentially distributed to the lower lung, this can cause V̇/Q̇ mismatching and desaturation.

It's easy to remember which way round this is as it is obvious that blood will preferentially perfuse the dependent lung under the influence of gravity. In our natural state, e.g. asleep in bed on our side, nature would not invent a system that would worsen oxygenation – so the air must also flow into the dependent lung to increase V̇/Q̇ matching. A practical application of this principle can be seen in ITU when we see patients improve/desaturate as they are turned and the good/bad lung is preferentially ventilated.

Summary of distribution (%) of ventilation under anaesthesia in the lateral position:

	Dependent Lung	Non-dependent Lung
Awake	60%	40%
GA spontaneous breathing	45%	55%
GA IPPV	40%	60%
Thoracotomy	30%	70%

CHAPTER 15

Baroreceptors and control of blood pressure

What types of baroreceptor are there?

Baroreceptors respond to stretch and are also known as stretch receptors. They are located within vessel walls and the cardiac chambers. They consist of sprayed, myelinated nerve endings, which form a reflex feedback mechanism involved in the regulation of blood pressure.

Baroreceptors may be classified as high pressure or low pressure:

➤ **High-pressure arterial baroreceptors:** Located within the walls of the aortic arch and carotid sinus (a small dilatation of the internal carotid artery just above its bifurcation). Due to their proximity to blood leaving the heart these receptors are well positioned to control perfusion pressures to the coronary and cerebral circulations. They are involved in the rapid short-term control of blood pressure.

➤ **Low-pressure baroreceptors:** Located in the chambers of the heart, large systemic veins and the pulmonary vasculature. These receptors bring about changes in blood volume and are involved in the slower and sustained control of blood pressure.

How do the high-pressure baroreceptors work?

➤ The sprayed nerve endings of the aortic arch baroreceptors discharge impulses along the vagus nerve while the carotid sinus baroreceptors discharge impulses along the glossopharyngeal nerve to the vasomotor and cardio-inhibitory centres located in the medulla.

➤ As blood pressure rises, the rate of discharge along these nerves increases, leading to a reduction in sympathetic outflow and increase in parasympathetic transmission. The consequent reduction in blood vessel tone, heart rate and contractility leads to a reduction in blood pressure (MAP = SV × HR × SVR). Conversely, the rate of discharge decreases with reductions in blood pressure leading to increased sympathetic outflow.

➤ As this system relies on neural transmission it is extremely fast and is responsible for the beat-to-beat control of blood pressure. For example, these baroreceptors mediate the bradycardia that is sometimes observed in patients following administration of a bolus dose of vasopressor such as phenylephrine.

What reflexes are elicited by a rapid fall in blood pressure, e.g. sudden 2 L blood loss?

The physiological response involves cardiovascular, neurohumoral and renal compensatory mechanisms:

➤ Baroreceptor reflex activation – immediate response
  • Reduced baroreceptor (aortic arch and carotid sinus) input due to reduced vessel stretch leads to reduced afferent discharge in glossopharyngeal and vagus nerves. Cardio-inhibitory centre is inhibited while the vasomotor centre is activated, leading to reduced parasympathetic activity and increased sympathetic activity resulting in increased force of cardiac contraction, tachycardia and increased SVR.

➤ Cardiovascular
  • Redistribution of cardiac output from skin, muscle and viscera to brain and heart.

➤ Hypothalamic – Pituitary – Adrenal responses
  • Increased ADH secretion from the posterior pituitary, leading to water conservation.
  • Increased adrenal release of noradrenaline, adrenaline and cortisol via sympathetic nervous system activation.
➤ Starling's forces
  • Favour interstitial fluid movement into the circulation through fall in intravascular hydrostatic pressure and rise in oncotic pressure.
➤ Renin – Angiotensin – Aldosterone system
  • Fall in renal blood flow detected by juxtaglomerular apparatus, leads to release of renin and its subsequent conversion to angiotensin 2, which causes vasoconstriction and stimulates the release of aldosterone.
  • Aldosterone increases sodium and water reabsorption at the distal convoluted tubules, thereby expanding plasma volume.

What is the Bainbridge reflex?
A rapid increase in venous return to the heart (e.g. rapid IV fluid bolus) may lead to activation of atrial stretch receptors resulting in an increase in heart rate.

What is the Bezold-Jarisch reflex?
Ventricular ischaemia (e.g. myocardial infarction) results in activation of ventricular receptors, which leads to bradycardia and hypotension.

Describe the physiological control of blood pressure
Blood pressure regulation occurs not only from beat to beat but also in the longer term over months to years. Mean arterial pressure is the product of cardiac output (heart rate × stroke volume) and systemic vascular resistance.

$$MAP = CO \times SVR$$

➤ **Short-term regulation:** Mediated largely by the arterial and cardiac baroreceptors and the vasomotor centre in the nucleus tractus solitarius, which ultimately alter the balance between parasympathetic and sympathetic discharge, thereby altering heart rate, stroke volume and systemic vascular resistance.
➤ **Long-term regulation:** Mediated by neurohumoral, renal, metabolic, race and genetic factors. The following factors may all chronically affect long-term blood pressure:
  • sodium intake
  • atrial natriuretic peptide
  • bradykinin
  • nitric oxide
  • glucocorticoids
  • renal function
  • psychological stress
  • obesity – with a possible link to insulin resistance
  • atherosclerosis
  • renin – angiotensin – aldosterone system.

CHAPTER 16

Cardiac cycle

Describe the pressure changes that occur during the cardiac cycle
This is a core topic and a common examination question. Make sure you are able to draw
the cardiac cycle and explain the pressure changes and events during each of the five phases.

Describe the five phases of the cardiac cycle
Phase 1: atrial contraction.
Phase 2: ventricular isovolumetric contraction.
Phase 3: ventricular ejection.
Phase 4: ventricular isovolumetric relaxation.
Phase 5: passive ventricular filling.

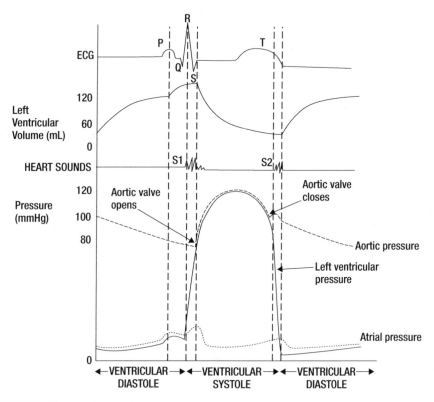

FIGURE 1.24 The cardiac cycle

CHAPTER 17

Coronary circulation

Describe the coronary circulation
➤ The arterial blood supply to the heart comes from the right coronary artery (RCA) and the left coronary artery (LCA), which arise from the anterior and posterior aortic sinuses respectively.
➤ The RCA supplies the right atrium, right ventricle, sinoatrial node and in 90% of people also the atrioventricular node.
➤ The LCA divides into the left anterior descending (LAD) artery and the left circumflex (LCx) artery and supplies the left atrium, left ventricle and most of the interventricular septum.
➤ In 30% of the population the LCA and RCA supply an equal share of the blood but in 50% the RCA is the dominant vessel.
➤ Venous drainage occurs predominantly via the coronary sinus. This receives blood from the great cardiac vein (draining the anterior aspect of the heart) and the middle cardiac vein (draining the posterior aspect of the heart). In addition there are other vessels that drain directly into the heart chambers including the thebesian veins, which contribute towards true shunt.

What is autoregulation?
Autoregulation refers to the intrinsic ability of an organ to maintain a constant blood flow despite a varying perfusion pressure. The heart, kidney and brain are all examples of organs that exhibit this property.

How is coronary blood flow autoregulated?
The heart can autoregulate its blood supply at coronary perfusion pressures (CoPP) between 60 and 180 mmHg. Outside this range, the coronary circulation becomes pressure-dependent.
Autoregulation occurs via a combination of the following mechanisms:
➤ **Metabolic:** During periods of increased myocardial activity, local tissue hypoxia and increased metabolic waste products like H^+, K^+ adenosine and CO_2 cause vasodilatation of the coronary vessels, thereby increasing coronary blood flow.
➤ **Myogenic:** When the pressure within a small artery or arteriole is increased, the smooth muscle within these vessels automatically constricts, thereby reducing blood flow. The reverse happens when the pressure within such vessels falls.
➤ **Endothelial:** Vascular endothelium produces various vasoactive substances including nitric oxide (NO), endothelium derived relaxing factor (EDRF) and prostacyclin (PGI_2), all of which produce vasodilatation; conversely endothelin and thromboxane A_2 produce vasoconstriction. When endothelium is damaged (e.g. atherosclerotic plaques or ischaemia) the production of these vasoactive substances is reduced, making coronary vessels prone to vasospasm and platelet aggregation.
➤ **Autonomic:** ANS exerts a weak effect on the coronary circulation. α-adrenergic receptor stimulation causes vasoconstriction while β-adrenergic and vagal stimulation leads to vasodilatation of coronary vessels.

➤ **Hormonal:** Vasoactive hormones require an intact endothelium in order to produce their effect. Atrial natriuretic peptide causes vasodilatation while vasopressin and angiotensin II cause vasoconstriction.

What factors affect myocardial oxygen supply?

Myocardial oxygen supply is determined by coronary blood flow and the arterial oxygen content (CaO_2).

➤ **Determinants of coronary blood flow:**

- **Coronary perfusion pressure** (CoPP = Aortic pressure – Intraventricular pressure). During systole the CoPP of the left ventricle can equal zero (or less) and therefore coronary bloods flow only occurs during diastole.

   In systole:

   LVCoPP = [SBP–LVESP]= [120 mmHg – 120 mmHg]= 0 mmHg

   In diastole:

   LVCoPP = [DBP–LVEDP] = [70 mmHg – 10 mmHg] = 60 mmHg.

   However, the coronary blood flow to both atria and the right ventricle occurs throughout the cardiac cycle.

   In systole:

   RVCoPP = [SBP – RVESP] = [120–25] = 95 mmHg

   In diastole:

   RVCoPP = [DBP – RVEDP] = [70–5] = 65 mmHg.

- **Perfusion time:** As the heart rate increases, the diastolic time and therefore the coronary perfusion time, especially to the left ventricle, is reduced.
- **Coronary vessel patency:** Atherosclerotic vessels are stenosed and have a reduced blood flow (as indicated by the Hagen-Poiseuille formula).
- **Coronary vessel diameter:** The wider the diameter, the greater the blood flow (hence the administration of GTN in angina).
- **Blood viscosity:** Haematocrit is a major determinant of blood viscosity and from the Hagen-Poiseuille formula it can be seen that as viscosity increases, flow decreases. However, as haematocrit decreases, so does the oxygen-carrying capacity of blood.

➤ **Determinants of arterial oxygen content:**

   $CaO_2 = [Hb \times Sats \times 1.34] + [PaO_2 \times 0.023]$

   From this equation it can be seen that the only parameters we can manipulate are the Hb and the PaO_2 (*see* Chapter 4, 'Oxygen transport', for full explanation of above equation).

What are the major determinants of myocardial oxygen consumption?

➤ The heart has the highest oxygen consumption per tissue mass of any organ in the body, requiring 10 mL O_2/min/100 g at rest and 70 mL/min/100 g during heavy exercise (the kidney uses 5 mL/min/100 g while the brain uses 3 mL/min/100 g). As a result, the heart receives 5% of the cardiac output, giving it a coronary blood flow of 250 mL/min.

➤ In order to support such high oxygen consumption, the heart at rest extracts approximately 70% of its coronary blood oxygen content (remember that the rest of the body only extracts on average 25% of its arterial O_2 content). Therefore, during periods of increased mechanical activity the only way the heart can meet its increased oxygen consumption is by increasing its coronary blood flow.

➤ Factors which determine myocardial oxygen consumption include heart rate, contractility, afterload, tissue mass and temperature (cold cardioplegic solutions are used during cardiopulmonary bypass surgery to reduce myocardial oxygen consumption and minimise risk of ischaemia).

CHAPTER 18

Exercise

The physiological response to exercise involves primarily cardio-respiratory and metabolic adaptations. The exact physiological response is determined not only by the intensity and duration of exercise but also by the underlying level of fitness of the individual.

Describe the physiological changes that occur in response to exercise

In healthy individuals, predictable physiological changes occur during exercise.

At rest, oxygen consumption is approximately 250 mL/min. During strenuous exercise oxygen consumption may rise to over 4000 mL/min. This massive increase in oxygen consumption requires a cardio-respiratory response to increase oxygen delivery.

Respiratory changes:

➤ On initiation of exercise, minute ventilation increases dramatically from a basal rate of approximately 5 L/min to over 20 L/min via a combination of increase in respiratory rate and tidal volume. This initial increase is thought to occur in response to afferent impulses from proprioceptors in muscle.

➤ As exercise progresses, minute ventilation continues to rise linearly with work rate and may reach in excess of 150 L/min.

➤ Oxygen consumption also increases linearly with work rate, until a certain point known as $\dot{V}O_2$ max, at which point it becomes constant. Any increase in work rate above $\dot{V}O_2$ max can only occur via anaerobic glycolysis. $\dot{V}O_2$ max is the best and most reproducible index of cardiopulmonary fitness.

➤ Minimal changes occur in arterial pH, $PaCO_2$ and PaO_2 during exercise.

Cardiovascular changes:

➤ Cardiac output increases in response to a rise in heart rate and augmentation of stroke volume through increased force of systolic contraction. These chronotropic and inotropic effects on the heart are the result of activation of the sympathetic nervous system. In trained athletes, the left ventricle hypertrophies and a resting bradycardia is often present. Trained athletes may achieve cardiac outputs in excess of 30 L/min during exercise.

➤ Muscle blood flow is increased during exercise as a consequence of accumulation of metabolites such as adenosine and potassium. Consequently, SVR is reduced. Oxygen extraction by the muscle is also increased during exercise.

➤ The oxyhaemoglobin dissociation curve is shifted to the right because of the reduced local pH in exercising muscle and the increased temperature.

➤ Blood is also redistributed to the skin to enable heat loss.

What metabolic changes occur during exercise?

A diagram may be useful to provide an overview of metabolism:

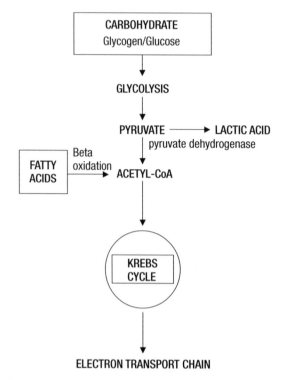

FIGURE 1.25 Overview of metabolism

➤ ATP is the most important energy substrate and is essential for muscle contraction. Aerobic metabolism is more efficient than anaerobic metabolism.

➤ On initiation of exercise, stored ATP provides the energy for muscle contraction. However, the store of ATP is small and therefore re-synthesis of ATP during exercise is essential. ATP is re-synthesised from glycogen and glucose initially and then from fatty acids.

➤ Through the glycolytic pathway glucose and glycogen are converted to produce two molecules of pyruvate. If oxygen is available, pyruvate is converted to acetyl-CoA and enters the Krebs cycle to supply the electron transport chain. This yields 39 mols of ATP per molecule of glycogen.

➤ If, however, oxygen is not present, pyruvate cannot be converted to acetyl-CoA; instead pyruvate forms lactic acid via lactate dehydrogenase, and this generates 3 mols of ATP per molecule of glycogen.

➤ As glycogen stores become depleted during prolonged exercise, metabolism switches increasingly to fatty acids. If fat is fully oxidised via the Krebs cycle it leads to the generation of 129 mols of ATP. However, the rate of ATP re-synthesis from fat is too slow to be of great importance during high intensity exercise such as sprinting but is important in endurance exercise.

➤ Under normal circumstances protein metabolism does not contribute to ATP generation because it is an essential structural component of the body. However, in extreme conditions (e.g. ultra marathon runners or starvation) protein can be used to generate ATP.

What is the anaerobic threshold?

When the metabolic demands of exercise begin to exceed oxygen delivery to the muscles, anaerobic metabolism ensues. Above the anaerobic threshold, blood lactate levels increase and the lactate to pyruvate ratio also rises. The anaerobic threshold typically occurs between 45% and 65% of the $\dot{V}O_2$ max in healthy untrained individuals and generally does not exceed 80% even in endurance-trained athletes.

Training can result in an increase in both $\dot{V}O_2$ max and anaerobic threshold.

What is the respiratory exchange ratio (RER)?

➤ The RER is the ratio of CO_2 production to O_2 consumption:

$$RER = \dot{V}CO_2/\dot{V}O_2$$

➤ The RER represents the metabolic exchange of gases in the body's tissues and is dependent in part on the predominant fuel (carbohydrate vs. fat) used for cellular metabolism.

➤ At rest and with early exercise, the $\dot{V}CO_2$ curve runs slightly below the $\dot{V}O_2$ curve (RER 0.8) but once the anaerobic threshold is passed, additional non-metabolic CO_2 is produced, resulting in a steep rise in $\dot{V}CO_2$ and an accompanying rise in the RER, ultimately exceeding 1.0.

CHAPTER 19

Starvation

Many patients admitted to hospital experience poor nutritional intake either as a direct result of their disease process or because of poor oral intake. Starvation has clinically important effects on the body and the physiological and biochemical adaptations that occur in response to starvation lend themselves to an excellent examination question.

Think of the physiology of starvation as the body's metabolic adaptations to reduce protein breakdown.

What stores of energy does a 70 kg male possess?
Energy is stored as carbohydrate, protein and fat.
➤ 1600 kcal as glycogen
➤ 24 000 kcal in mobilisable protein
➤ 135 000 kcal in triacylglycerols

[kcal is an abbreviation for kilocalorie, which is equivalent to 1 calorie, or about 4.185 kJ (kilojoules)]

What are the 24-hour energy requirements of a 70 kg male at rest?
1600–2000 kcal per 24 hours (this may rise to 6000 kcal with stress).

If there is no energy intake, how does the body adapt?
➤ Carbohydrate reserves (glycogen) only last approximately 24 hours. Despite the exhaustion of glycogen, blood glucose levels are maintained. The brain cannot tolerate low blood glucose for even short periods and so the first priority of metabolism in starvation is to provide sufficient glucose to both the brain and red blood cells, both of which are absolutely dependent on this fuel source.
➤ A lot of energy is stored in triacylglycerols. However, fatty acids cannot be converted into glucose because acetyl-CoA cannot be converted into pyruvate and so the only other source of glucose is amino acids derived from protein breakdown (i.e. muscle breakdown). Yet survival is dependent on maintaining protein and muscle. Thus the second priority of metabolism in starvation is to preserve protein and so the body shifts its primary fuel source from glucose to fatty acids and ketones.

What adaptations occur during the first 24 hours of starvation?
➤ As blood glucose levels begin to fall, insulin secretion is reduced and its counter-regulatory hormone glucagon is secreted, leading to mobilisation of triacylglycerols in fat and gluconeogenesis by the liver.
➤ Concentrations of acetyl-CoA and citrate rise, which reduces glycolysis.
➤ Muscle uptake of glucose reduces secondary to the lack of insulin and therefore muscle also shifts to fatty acid use for fuel.
➤ Pyruvate is no longer converted into acetyl-CoA and therefore pyruvate, lactate and alanine are exported to the liver for conversion into glucose.

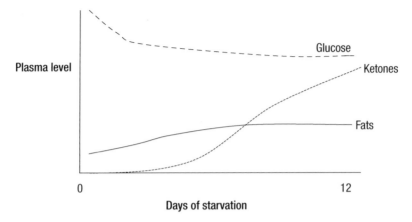

GRAPH 1.26 Plasma glucose, ketone and fatty acid levels in starvation

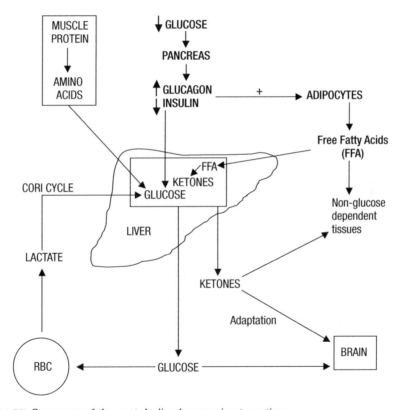

FIGURE 1.27 Summary of the metabolic changes in starvation

What adaptations occur 72 hours into starvation?
➤ The most important metabolic change is the hepatic production of large amounts of ketone bodies (acetoacetate and 3-hydroxybutarate) from acetyl-CoA.
➤ The occurs because gluconeogenesis depletes the supply of oxaloacetate, which is essential for acetyl-CoA to enter the Krebs cycle, and therefore instead the acetyl-CoA is used for ketogenesis.

➤ The brain now begins to utilise acetoacetate (ketone body) for 30% of its energy requirements, i.e. adaptation has occurred.

➤ The heart is also able to utilise ketones as an energy source.

What adaptations occur several weeks into starvation?

➤ Ketones now become the major fuel source for the brain (>70%).

➤ The effective conversion of fatty acids into ketones by the liver and their subsequent use by the brain markedly diminishes the need for glucose and therefore reduces muscle breakdown.

➤ The duration of starvation compatible with life is determined by the size of the triacylglycerol stores.

➤ **Early starvation** – reduction in energy expenditure, glycogen stores used within 24 hours, use of alternative fuels such as ketones to minimise protein wasting.

➤ **Late starvation** – fatty acids, ketones and glycerol provide all of the energy requirements for the body, except for the brain and red blood cells, which still require a glucose source.

CHAPTER 20

Nausea and vomiting

Nausea and vomiting are hazards of both general and regional anaesthesia. Post-operative nausea and vomiting (PONV) is one of the most distressing complications following surgery and anaesthesia, and in some studies it has been found to be as distressing as pain.

Define nausea and vomiting
➤ **Nausea** is the sensation of the need to vomit.
➤ **Vomiting** is the involuntary, forceful expulsion of gastric contents via the mouth.

Describe the physiology of vomiting
The physiology of vomiting is complex with multiple afferent and efferent pathways; an overview is helpful:

The chemoreceptor trigger zone (CTZ) lies in the floor of the fourth ventricle in the area postrema and is functionally outside of the blood brain barrier. It contains dopamine (D_2) and serotonin (5-HT_3) receptors. The CTZ provides efferent input to the vomiting centre, which is located in the medulla. The vestibular system, peripheral pain pathways, intestinal chemoreceptors and the cerebral cortex all provide direct afferent input to the vomiting centre via cranial nerves VIII, IX and X.

Describe the process of vomiting
Vomiting is an involuntary reflex and may be divided into two phases, a pre-ejection phase and ejection phase.
➤ **Pre-ejection phase:**
  • nausea
  • sympathetic stimulation – tachycardia, tachypnoea, sweating
  • parasympathetic stimulation – salivation, upper and lower oesophageal sphincters relax; giant retrograde contraction.
➤ **Ejection phase:**
  • respiration temporarily ceases mid-inspiration
  • hyoid and larynx raised to open crico-oesphageal sphincter
  • glottis closes
  • soft palate elevates to close off the nasopharynx
  • contraction of the diaphragm and abdominal muscles results in a rise in intra-abdominal pressure
  • gastro-oesophageal sphincter opens
  • ejection of gastric contents.

What are the potential complications of vomiting?
Vomiting may result in potentially life-threatening complications:
➤ aspiration (particularly if GCS is obtunded)
➤ wound dehiscence
➤ electrolyte imbalance (loss of hydrogen, potassium and chloride)

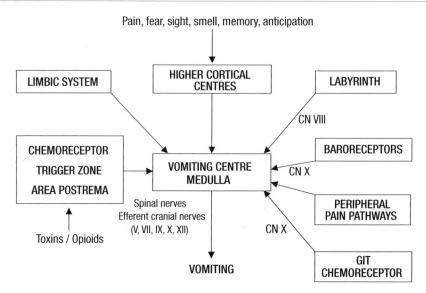

FIGURE 1.28 Overview of nausea and vomiting

➤ dehydration
➤ elevated intraocular and intracranial pressure.

What are the main risk factors for PONV?
Divide the answer into patient, anaesthetic and surgical factors.

Patient factors
➤ Female gender
➤ Non-smoker
➤ Previous PONV
➤ History of motion sickness

Anaesthetic factors
➤ Use of N_2O
➤ Use of opiates
➤ Use of etomidate
➤ Use of neostigmine
➤ Hypotension

Surgical factors
➤ Middle ear surgery
➤ Ophthalmic surgery (especially squint correction surgery)
➤ Gynaecology surgery

CHAPTER 21

Liver physiology

The liver is a complex organ with multiple functions and as such plays a key role in home-ostasis; its importance is best illustrated in acute liver failure.

There are a number of aspects of hepatic physiology that may be covered in an exam question and this answer should provide you with the pertinent key points.

Describe the anatomy of the liver
➤ Adult liver weight is 1800–2000 g.
➤ Divided into right and left hemi-liver plus caudate lobe.
➤ Histological unit of the liver is the lobule. Lobules are hexagonal in shape and have several portal triads located at their periphery.
➤ Portal triad is composed of hepatic artery, portal vein and bile duct.
➤ The central vein (branch of hepatic vein) is present in the centre of the lobule, surrounded by hepatocytes.
➤ Sinusoids traverse the lobule, draining blood from the peripheral portal triads to the central vein.
➤ Sinusoids also contain Kuppfer cells, part of the reticuloendothelial system.
➤ Hepatocytes produce bile which is excreted into the hepatic ducts of the portal triad via the bile cannaliculi.
➤ Functional unit of the liver is the acinus, a diamond-shaped area of the liver supplied by a terminal branch of the portal vein and of the hepatic artery and drained by a terminal branch of the bile duct.

What are hepatic zones?
The liver acinus is divided into zones 1 to 3. The portal triad is composed of the hepatic artery, portal vein and bile duct. It is the portal triad that forms the centre of the acinus and as such forms zone 1. Blood becomes progressively poorer in oxygen and nutrients from zone 1 to zone 3 (i.e. zone 3 represents the microcirculatory periphery).
➤ **Zone 1** – Hepatocytes close to the portal triad. Surrounding blood is rich in oxygen and nutrients. Mitochondria-rich cells are present which are suited to oxidative metabolism and glycogen synthesis.
➤ **Zone 3** – Hepatocytes at the periphery of the acinus, which receive blood that has already undergone exchange of gases and metabolites with cells in zones 1 and 2. Zone 3 is rich in smooth endoplasmic reticulum and cytochrome P450, making this the key region for drug and toxin biotransformation. It is also this zone that is most at risk of cellular damage during circulatory disturbances.

Describe the blood supply to the liver
➤ The liver is an extremely vascular organ, receiving a blood supply of 100 mL/kg/min (approximately 1800 mL/min).
➤ It has a dual blood supply, receiving approximately 70% of its blood flow from the portal vein and 30% from the hepatic artery.

➤ The portal vein is formed by the union of the splenic vein and superior mesenteric vein and thus carries blood from the gastrointestinal tract to the liver.
➤ The hepatic artery is a branch of the celiac artery.
➤ However, hepatic portal vein blood only has an oxygen saturation of approximately 70%, thus it provides only approximately 40% of the liver's oxygen requirements.
➤ The hepatic artery provides approximately 60% of the liver's oxygen requirements.
➤ Normal hepatic oxygen extraction is less than 50%. However, this can increase in response to increased oxygen demand.

What factors affect blood flow to the liver?
➤ Blood flow through the hepatic artery is autoregulated (maintenance of constant flow despite changes in mean arterial pressure) down to a mean arterial pressure of approximately 60 mmHg, below which flow is pressure-dependent.
➤ In contrast, blood flow through the portal vein is passive and dependent upon splanchnic blood flow.
➤ Therefore, only the arterial component of hepatic blood flow is controllable.
➤ The hepatic arterial blood flow is under intrinsic and extrinsic control.
➤ **Intrinsic control of hepatic arterial blood flow:**
  • **Myogenic response:** As the mean arterial pressure rises, the hepatic artery constricts to maintain a constant blood flow and vice versa.
  • **Hepatic arterial buffer response** (arteriovenous reciprocity): As hepatic portal venous flow changes, the hepatic artery vasoconstricts or vasodilates reciprocally in order to maintain overall constant hepatic blood flow.
➤ **Extrinsic control of hepatic blood flow:**
  • **Sympathetic nervous system:** stimulation results in hepatic arterial vasoconstriction.
  • **Drugs:** volatiles and noradrenaline reduce hepatic blood flow.
  • **General anaesthesia and spinal anaesthesia:** both reduce hepatic blood flow.
  • **Surgical handling of the liver:** reduces hepatic blood flow.

Classify and discuss the functions of the liver
Think of a patient with hepatic failure, who may exhibit the following symptoms or signs because of loss of hepatic function: jaundice, encephalopathy, coagulopathy, ascites, raised intracranial pressure, hypoglycaemia, renal dysfunction, loss of vascular tone and immunosuppression.
➤ **Biotransformation:** The liver plays a key role in the biotransformation of drugs, chemicals and toxins via the cytochrome P450 electron transport chain.
  • **Phase 1 reactions** (Hydrolysis/Oxidation/Reduction) – provide a reactive group for subsequent phase 2 reactions. They generally reduce the activity of a drug but may sometimes produce a toxic or active intermediate. If, following phase 1 reactions, the product is water-soluble, it will not require further phase 2 reactions but will be renally excreted.
  • **Phase 2 reactions** (Glucuronidation/Acetylation/Sulphonation/Methylation) – conjugation of phase 1 products via the above chemical processes to increase water solubility allowing renal or biliary excretion of the compound.
  • **Factors determining hepatic clearance:**
    – proportion of unbound drug in the plasma (cf. highly protein-bound drugs)
    – rate of drug presentation to the liver (i.e. flow limited) – important for drugs with high first-pass metabolism, e.g. morphine and lignocaine

- rate of enzymatic breakdown (i.e. capacity-limited) – important for drugs with low first-pass metabolism, e.g. diazepam and warfarin
- may be increased or decreased by hepatic enzyme inducers or inhibitors respectively
- hepatic function, e.g. affected by disease processes such as cirrhosis.
➤ **Synthetic function:** Synthesis of albumin, immunoglobulins, clotting factors (all except factor VIII), haptoglobin, C-reactive protein and anti-thrombin III.
➤ **Metabolic functions:**
  - **Carbohydrates** – the liver maintains blood glucose concentrations via glycogenesis, gluconeogenesis and glycogenolysis.
  - **Proteins** – synthesises, transaminates or deaminates proteins. Converts ammonia into the less toxic urea.
  - **Lipids** – synthesises cholesterol and triglycerides.
  - **Ketone bodies** – produces acetoacetate and β-hydroxybutarate.
  - **Vitamins** – activates vitamin D.
➤ **Digestive functions:** The liver produces bile. Bile is primarily utilised for the emulsification of dietary lipids to allow their absorption. In addition, bile is required for the absorption of fat-soluble vitamins A, D, E and K.
➤ **Storage functions:**
  - The liver stores approximately 100 g of glycogen.
  - Vitamins A, D, E, K.
  - Copper.
  - Iron (as ferritin).
➤ **Capacitance function:** At any one time the liver can hold as much as 15% of the circulating volume and therefore can act as a large blood reservoir. Approximately half of this blood can be returned to the circulation during periods of sympathetic stimulation.
➤ **Immunological function:** Kupffer cells form part of the reticuloendothelial system and have the function of removal of old erythrocytes, bacteria and other antigens via phagocytosis.

Give examples of some liver function tests
➤ **Alanine and aspartate aminotransferases (ALT and AST)**
  - Released into the blood following hepatocelluar damage.
  - Serum level does not correlate with extent of liver injury.
  - ALT more liver-specific than AST.
➤ **Indicators of biliary tract disease**
  - Elevated conjugated bilirubin.
  - Elevated alkaline phosphatase (ALP) and gamma-glutamyl transferase (GGT).
➤ **Indicators of hepatic synthetic function**
  - All clotting factors are synthesised by the liver except factor VIII.
  - Prothrombin time (PT) indirectly determines the amount of available clotting factors and is therefore used to assess synthetic function.
  - Serum albumin is difficult to interpret in the setting of critical illness because of renal and gastrointestinal losses. However, it will be reduced in chronic liver disease.

CHAPTER 22

Gastric regulation

Describe what happens in the GI tract when a meal is anticipated

There are three main phases of gastric regulation:
➤ cephalic phase
➤ gastric phase
➤ intestinal phase.

Cephalic phase

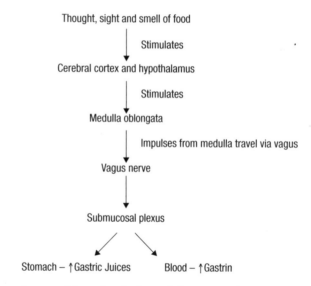

Thought, sight and smell of food

Stimulates

Cerebral cortex and hypothalamus

Stimulates

Medulla oblongata

Impulses from medulla travel via vagus

Vagus nerve

Submucosal plexus

Stomach – ↑ Gastric Juices   Blood – ↑ Gastrin

These reflexes are decreased by stimulation of the sympathetic nervous system with, for example, pain, fear and anxiety.

Gastric phase
➤ As food and fluid enter the stomach, stretch and chemoreceptors are activated.
➤ This leads to a further increase in gastric secretions and increases peristalsis.
➤ The tone of the lower oesophageal sphincter is increased to prevent reflux of acid.
➤ Once the pH has reached 2 then gastrin begins to exert a negative feedback to inhibit further acid secretion.

Intestinal phase
This begins when chyme (food mixed with gastric juices) enters the duodenum, causing the secretion of three main gut hormones:
➤ gastric inhibitory peptide (GIP), which inhibits further gastric secretions and motility
➤ secretin, which inhibits further gastric secretions
➤ cholecystokinin (CCK), which inhibits stomach emptying.

Describe the function of these gut hormones
There are four main hormones involved: gastrin, GIP, secretin and CCK.

TABLE 1.29 Functions of gut hormones

Hormone	Release stimulated by:	Actions
Gastrin	Cephalic phase	↑ Secretion of gastric juices
	Stomach distension	↑ Motility
	Proteins in stomach	Encourages growth of mucosa
	↑ pH of chyme in stomach	Constricts LOS
		Relaxes pyloric and ileocaecal sphincters
GIP	Fatty acids in small intestine	↑ Insulin release
		Inhibits secretion of gastric juices
		Slows gastric emptying
Secretin	Acidic chyme in small intestine	Stimulates contraction of gallbladder to release bile
		Stimulates release of pancreatic enzymes
		Augments effect of CCK
CCK	Amino acids in small intestine	Stimulates contraction of gallbladder to release bile
	Fatty acids in small intestine	Stimulates release of pancreatic enzymes
		Induces feeling of satiety
		Inhibits gastric emptying
		Enhances actions of secretin

Describe the sphincters present in the gastrointestinal tract
A sphincter is a structure, usually made up of circular muscle, which surrounds the opening of a hollow organ or body, and constricts to close it. Sphincters can be anatomical, where they are clearly different from the surrounding tissue, e.g. the anus, or functional where the histological distinction is not so clear, e.g. lower oesophageal sphincter. Sphincters can be under voluntary or involuntary control. There are many sphincters in the gastrointestinal tract:
➤ upper oesophageal
➤ lower oesophageal
➤ pyloric
➤ ileocaecal
➤ sphincter of Oddi
➤ anus.

Upper oesophageal sphincter: This is at the level of the C5–6 vertebrae and is made up of the cricopharyngeal part of the inferior pharyngeal constrictor muscle. It is under conscious control and in its resting state it is usually constricted to avoid air being drawn into the stomach during breathing.

Lower oesophageal sphincter (also called the 'cardiac' sphincter): This is a functional sphincter, found at the junction between the non-keratinised squamous epithelium of the oesophagus and the simple columnar epithelium of the stomach. Its function is to prevent reflux of the acidic stomach contents into the oesophagus and so it is constricted at rest, and has a pressure of 15–20 mmHg. The sphincter opens ahead of peristalsis during the process of swallowing to allow food and fluid to enter the stomach. It is supplied by the vagus nerve.

'**Barrier pressure**' describes the difference between LOS pressure and intragastric pressure. The closer the barrier pressure is to zero, the more likely it is that reflux will occur. So, reducing LOS tone (*see* causes in Figure 1.30, on the following page) or increasing intragastric pressure (e.g. pregnancy, full stomach, abdominal distension) make reflux more likely.

Pyloric sphincter: This is an anatomical sphincter found at the junction of the stomach and duodenum. Its ring of muscle relaxes to allow chyme to pass out of the stomach. It is supplied by the coeliac ganglion.

Ileocaecal sphincter: An anatomical sphincter found at the junction of the small and large bowel. It prevents reflux of colonic material into ileum.

Sphincter of Oddi: This is a ring of muscle that surrounds the bile and pancreatic ducts as they emerge into the lumen of the duodenum, about halfway down its length. The sphincter controls the release of bile and pancreatic enzymes into the duodenum.

Anus: The gastrointestinal tract ends in a pouch called the rectum, where faeces are stored prior to defecation. At the exit of the rectum is the anorectal junction, a voluntary sphincter that is made up of an internal and external ring of muscle. The internal anal sphincter is supplied by the hypogastric plexus. It is involuntary and will relax in response to stretching. The external anal sphincter is voluntary and supplied by the inferior rectal nerves.

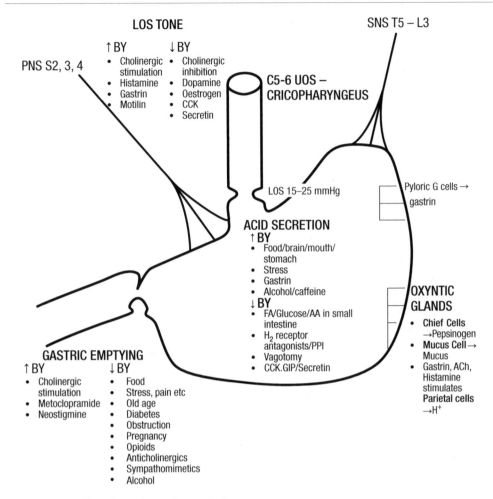

FIGURE 1.30 Overview of gastric regulation

PNS	Parasympathetic nervous system
SNS	Sympathetic nervous system
UOS	Upper oesophageal sphincter
LOS	Lower oesophageal sphincter
FA	Fatty acids
AA	Amino acids
PPI	Proton pump inhibitors

CHAPTER 23

Total parenteral nutrition

Questions on parenteral nutrition have appeared in the primary examination, albeit rarely as the topic lends itself more towards the final examination. Nevertheless, as doctors who may be involved in prescribing total parenteral nutrition (TPN) within the critical care setting, examiners would expect a basic understanding of the indications, nutritional content requirements and complications associated with this form of feeding.

Parenteral nutrition is by definition administered intravenously. TPN supplies all daily nutritional requirements to the patient. In general, because TPN solutions are concentrated and therefore have the potential to cause venous thrombosis of peripheral veins, a central venous catheter is usually required.

Indications for TPN

Where possible the enteral route should always be used in preference to parenteral nutrition. However, where this is not possible, TPN should be considered.

➤ Anticipation of undernutrition (< 50% of metabolic requirements achieved enterally) for > 7 days.

➤ TPN may be indicated for severely undernourished patients unable to ingest large volumes of oral feed prior to surgery, radiation therapy or chemotherapy.

➤ Patients with disorders requiring complete gastrointestinal rest, e.g. ulcerative colitis/pancreatitis.

➤ Post-operative patients in whom enteral feeding has either not been possible or has failed after 5 days.

Nutritional content

TPN should be considered as a drug. Most hospitals in the UK now have a nutrition team comprising a physician, dietician and pharmacist, with the remit of reviewing patients with nutritional concerns and guiding safe use of parenteral nutrition.

Basic Adult Requirements for TPN

Water	30–40 mL/kg/day
Energy	Medical patient 30 kcal/kg/day
	Post-operative patient 30–45 kcal/kg/day
	Hypercatabolic patient 45–60 kcal/kg/day
Amino acids	Medical patient 1 g/day
	Post-operative patient 2 g/day
	Hypercatabolic patient 3 g/day
Essential fatty acids	
Minerals	Acetate/Calcium/Chloride/Copper/Magnesium
	Potassium/Selenium/Sodium/Zinc
Vitamins	A/D/E/K/C/Folic acid/Thiamine/Pyridoxine/Niacin

Basic TPN solutions are prepared using sterile techniques. Solutions may be modified based on laboratory results (e.g. electrolyte disturbances), underlying disorders, hypermetabolism or other factors. Commercially available lipid emulsions are often added to supply essential fatty acids and triglycerides; 20–30% of total calories are usually supplied as lipids. However, withholding lipids and their calories may help obese patients mobilise endogenous fat stores and increase their insulin sensitivity.

Electrolytes can be added to meet the patient's needs. Patients who have renal insufficiency and are not receiving haemofiltration or who have hepatic failure require solutions with reduced protein content and a higher percentage of essential amino acids. For patients with respiratory failure, a lipid emulsion must provide most of the non-protein calories in order to minimise CO_2 generation.

TPN administration and monitoring

Ideally, TPN should be administered through a dedicated port of a central venous line. Strict asepsis must be used during administration. The solution is commenced at 50% of the calculated requirements initially. Insulin may be required to maintain glycaemic control. Basic monitoring tests include daily weight, FBC, urea and electrolytes and liver function tests.

Complications

With close monitoring by a nutrition team complication rates should be < 5%, but may be related either to the central venous catheter (infection) or to the nutrition.

➤ **Volume overload** – may occur when high daily energy requirements require large volumes of fluid.
➤ **Glucose abnormalities** – hyperglycaemia may occur (less commonly hypoglycaemia) and thus regular blood glucose monitoring is essential.
➤ **Electrolyte disturbances** – primarily the clinically important electrolytes to be monitored are sodium, potassium, magnesium and phosphate.
➤ **Metabolic bone disease** – bone demineralisation develops in some patients receiving prolonged TPN (> 3 months). The only treatment is to discontinue the TPN temporarily or permanently.
➤ **Hepatic complications** – transient liver dysfunction on commencement of TPN is common, evidenced by increased hepatic transaminases, bilirubin and alkaline phosphatase. Delayed or persistent elevations may result from excess quantities of amino acids. The pathogenesis of the hepatic complications is not known.
➤ **Gallbladder complications** – include choletlithiasis and cholecystitis.
➤ **Refeeding syndrome** – is a relatively rare but potentially fatal complication of TPN and also a favoured examination question. The syndrome describes the severe hypophosphataemia and other metabolic complications which are seen in malnourished patients who then receive concentrated calories via TPN. The syndrome was first described in Japanese prisoners of war after the Second World War.

Refeeding syndrome usually occurs within 72 hours of commencement of feeding. The syndrome results from the sudden shift from fat to carbohydrate metabolism with a sudden rise in insulin secretion leading to an increased cellular uptake of phosphate, potassium, magnesium and glucose – thus serum levels of these electrolytes fall rapidly. The systemic consequences are acute cardiac failure, confusion, coma, convulsions and even death. Prevention of the syndrome involves identifying patients at risk – and introducing slow refeeding along with close monitoring and correction of electrolyte disturbances.

CHAPTER 24

Acid–base balance

A stable pH in body fluids is essential to maintain normal enzyme function, ion distribution and protein structure.

Homeostatic acid–base regulatory mechanisms aim to maintain a pH between 7.35 and 7.45 ([H⁺] of 45–35 nmol/L) via:

➤ buffers in tissue and blood
➤ excretion of acids by kidneys and lungs.

Normal acid–base balance relies on the following variables:

➤ pH ~ 7.40
➤ PCO_2 ~ 5.3 kPa (40 mmHg)
➤ HCO_3^- ~ 25 mmol/L

An acid–base disturbance occurs when at least two of these three variables are abnormal.

The primary change determines whether a disturbance is respiratory (alteration of PCO_2) or metabolic (alteration of the bicarbonate buffer system by means other than PCO_2).

Define the following:

➤ **Base:** proton acceptor, pH > 7.0
➤ **Acid:** proton donor, pH < 7.0
  The strength of an acid is defined by its ability to give up protons:
  • **Strong acid** (e.g. HCl): fully dissociates in solution
  • **Weak acid** (e.g. carbonic acid): does not fully dissociate, and, together with its conjugate base, it acts as an acid–base buffer system to resist a change in pH.
➤ **pH:** negative logarithm to the base 10 of the hydrogen ion concentration.
➤ **Acidosis:** a process where there is an excess of acid production.
➤ **Acidaemia:** occurs when the arterial pH < 7.35 or [H⁺] > 45 nmol/L.
➤ **Alkalosis:** a process where there is a reduced acid production.
➤ **Alkalaemia:** occurs when the arterial pH > 7.45 or [H⁺] < 35 nmol/L.
➤ **Standard bicarbonate:** plasma concentration of bicarbonate when arterial PCO_2 has been corrected to 5.3 kPa, haemoglobin is fully saturated and the body temperature is 37 °C. It represents what the actual bicarbonate would be after eliminating any respiratory component of acid–base disturbance.
➤ **Base excess (deficit):** the amount of acid or base required to restore 1 L of blood to normal pH at a $PaCO_2$ of 5.3 kPa and at body temperature. It is generally negative in acidosis and positive in alkalosis, and is a useful marker of severity of the metabolic component of acid base disturbances. The **Siggaard-Andersen nomogram** can be used to derive the base deficit and standard bicarbonate if the pH, PCO_2 and haemoglobin are known.

What compensatory mechanisms exist?

These aim to restore the pH towards normal, but do not reverse the primary change.

Correction occurs when all three variables (pH, PaO_2 and $PaCO_2$) are restored to normal levels.

➤ **Initial compensation** is by the **carbonic acid–bicarbonate buffer system** and occurs within 2 hours.
➤ **Renal compensation** is by:
  ● **Increased acid (H⁺) secretion and HCO₃⁻ retention** (reabsorption and regeneration) in the presence of a respiratory (and metabolic) acidosis.
  ● **Decreased acid (H⁺) secretion and HCO₃⁻ retention** (reabsorption and regeneration) in the presence of a respiratory (and metabolic) alkalosis.
     The generation of bicarbonate through urinary excretion of ammonium and phosphate restores the depleted HCO₃⁻ and buffer base reserves over 2–3 days.
➤ **Respiratory compensation** is by:
  ● **Hyperventilation** in the presence of a metabolic acidosis.
  ● **Hypoventilation** in the presence of a metabolic alkalosis.

TABLE 1.31 Mechanisms involved in acid–base balance

Primary disturbance	Compensatory bicarbonate change (mmol/L) per 1 kPa change in $PaCO_2$ from 5.3 kPa		Compensatory mechanism
	RISE	FALL	
Respiratory acidosis			Buffers
Acute	0.7		Renal: ↑ H⁺ secretion and HCO₃⁻ retention (note: the bicarbonate
Chronic	2.6		rise is 3–4 times more efficient in chronic disturbances)
Respiratory alkalosis			Buffers
Acute		1.3	Renal: ↓ H⁺ secretion and HCO₃⁻ retention (note: the bicarbonate
Chronic		4.0	fall is 3–4 times more efficient in chronic disturbances)
Metabolic acidosis		1.3	Buffers
			Respiratory: hyperventilation (min $PaCO_2$ of 1.3–1.9 kPa)
			Renal: ↑ acid secretion
Metabolic alkalosis	0.76		Buffers
			Respiratory: hypoventilation (max $PaCO_2$ of 7–8 kPa is reached within 24 hrs)
			Renal: ↓ acid secretion

Identify the abnormalities of these arterial blood gases: pH 7.0; $PaCO_2$ 7 kPa; PaO_2 7 kPa. What standard bicarbonate and base excess would you expect with these values?

Abnormality:	Acidaemia (pH < 7.4)
Process:	Acidosis (excess production of acid, in the form of CO_2)
Primary change:	Respiratory (↑ $PaCO_2$ and ↓ PaO_2, i.e. type 2 respiratory failure)
Acute vs. chronic:	Likely acute as uncompensated
Base excess/deficit:	Negative
Standard bicarbonate:	Low in acute setting, as slow renal compensation is incomplete

What would you expect the pH to be in patients with a chronically elevated $PaCO_2$ at 7 kPa?

In chronic respiratory acidosis, the renal compensatory mechanisms result in a chronic elevation of plasma bicarbonate, which in turn restores the pH to within the normal range. Typically, renal compensation is not complete, and the normal level of pH 7.4 is never reached.

How does metabolic compensation take place?

The increased $PaCO_2$ in the renal tubular cells results in an increased secretion of H^+ ions. Their secretion results in the following:

➤ Reabsorption of bicarbonate by the dissociation of carbonic acid.
➤ Regeneration of bicarbonate by the excretion of H^+ with ammonia and phosphate in urine.

Metabolic compensation takes place over 2–3 days.

Describe the physiological process accounting for the low pH

Respiratory acidosis is a consequence of hypoventilation or ventilation perfusion inequalities. The resulting elevated PCO_2 disrupts the ratio of HCO_3^- to PCO_2 and causes a drop in pH.

Comment on the PaO_2

This is lower than normal, suggesting either a problem with ventilation, diffusion, shunt or a ventilation-perfusion mismatch. Assuming the inspired concentration of oxygen is known, the alveolar partial pressure of oxygen can be calculated using the alveolar gas equation. The A–a gradient can then be worked out and type of hypoxia can be assessed, to help establish the cause.

CHAPTER 25

Buffers

What is the definition of a buffer?

An acid–base buffer solution resists a change of pH when an acid or base is added to it. It consists of a weak acid and its conjugate base (salt).

The general equation for a buffer system is:

HA (undissociated acid) ⇌ H⁺ (hydrogen ion) + A⁻ (conjugate base)

If H⁺ ions are added to the solution, the equilibrium shifts to the left, and the H⁺ are 'neutralised' by the conjugate base, minimising an increase in free [H⁺] and maintaining a constant pH.

If a base is added, H⁺ and OH⁻ react to form water, but more HA dissociates to maintain the [H⁺] constant, therefore the equation shifts to the right.

By applying the Law of Mass Action, $(K_a = [H^+][A^-]/[HA])$, the **Henderson–Hasselbalch equation** can be derived:

pH = pKa + log [conjugate base]/[acid]
pH = pKa + log [A⁻]/[HA]

and the dissociation constant (pKa) for a buffer system can be calculated.

What is a buffer titration curve?

➤ A titration curve is a plot of pH vs. the amount of acid or base added to a buffer solution (titration).

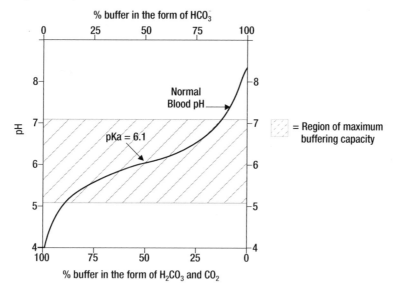

GRAPH 1.32 Buffer titration curve

➤ It is useful for determining dissociation constants (pK) of weak acids or bases.
➤ The pH is plotted on the y-axis and the buffer composition on the x-axis.
➤ For the bicarbonate and carbonic acid buffer system, on the left-hand side of the plot, most of the buffer is in the form of carbon dioxide or carbonic acid and, on the right-hand side of the plot, most of the buffer is in the form of bicarbonate ion.
➤ The curve is sigmoid in shape, with greater pH changes occurring at the extremes of buffer compositions.
➤ If acid is added, the pH decreases, and the buffer shifts towards a greater H_2CO_3 and CO_2 concentration.
➤ Conversely, as base is added, the pH increases and the buffer shifts towards a greater HCO_3^- concentration.
➤ The flatter part of the slope represents the area of greatest buffering capacity where a shift in the relative concentrations of bicarbonate and carbon dioxide produces only a small change in the pH of the solution.
➤ At the central point the pH is equal to the pKa (6.1) for the buffer.
➤ At the physiological blood pH of 7.4, small changes in the relative compositions cause a large change in pH.
➤ In order to maintain a constant pH, the body relies additionally on other buffer and organ systems.

What are the characteristics of an ideal buffer?
A good buffer solution must maintain a nearly constant pH when either acid or base is added. Two features render this possible:
➤ **Range of buffer** (defined as pH= pKa +/− 1): The buffer functions most effectively when its pKa is within one unit of the desired pH of the solution.
➤ **Buffering capacity:** This is defined by the ratio of the concentrations of weak acid to conjugate base, which must remain fairly constant, such that the addition of acid or base will not cause a change of pH.

What are the physiological buffer systems in the body?
TABLE 1.33 List of physiological buffers

Body compartment	Buffer system	(pKa)
Blood	Bicarbonate/carbonic acid	6.1
	Haemoglobin	7.8
	Plasma proteins	7.4
	Phosphate	6.8
Extracellular fluid	Bicarbonate/carbonic acid	
	Plasma proteins	
	Phosphate	
Intracellular fluid	Cellular proteins	
	Phosphate	
	Organic phosphates	
	Bicarbonate/carbonic acid	
Bone	Calcium carbonate	

Body compartment	Buffer system	(pKa)
Urine	Bicarbonate/carbonic acid	
	Phosphate (HPO_4^- /$H_2PO_4^{2-}$)	
	Ammonia (NH_3/NH_4^+)	9.0

The bicarbonate/carbonic acid buffer system:
➤ This is the most important system.
➤ Despite it having a low pKa (6.1) relative to blood pH, it is effective due to the ready excretion of carbonic acid in the form of CO_2 by the lungs, and the continuous regeneration of bicarbonate by the kidneys.
➤ It is more efficient at buffering acids since its efficiency increases as the pH falls.
➤ It is the main buffer system in the blood due to the abundance of plasma bicarbonate. The production of carbonic acid is catalysed by the enzyme carbonic anhydrase, which is present in red blood cells, but not in plasma.
The reaction for this buffer system is:

$$CO_2 + H_2O \rightleftharpoons H_2CO_3 \rightleftharpoons HCO_3^- + H^+$$

The Henderson–Hasselbalch equation for this buffer system is:

$$pH = 6.1 + \log [HCO_3^-]/[H_2CO_3]$$

and since H_2CO_3 is proportional to $PaCO_2$:

$$pH = 6.1 + \log [HCO_3^-]/0.225 \times PaCO_2$$

(0.225 is the solubility coefficient for $PaCO_2$ in kPa).

Haemoglobin
➤ Acts as a blood buffer by dissociation of the imidazole groups of its histidine residues (each molecule has 38 histidine residues).
➤ Deoxygenated haemoglobin is a better buffer (and weaker acid) than oxygenated haemoglobin because its imidazole groups dissociate less.
➤ It has six times the buffering capacity of plasma proteins.

Plasma and proteins
➤ These are effective buffers because both their carboxyl and free amino groups dissociate. Intracellular proteins are equally important.

Phosphate
➤ Plays a small role in the ECF, but is an important intracellular buffer due to its abundance and dissociation as follows: $H_2PO_4^- \rightleftharpoons HPO_4^{2-} + H^+$.

Urinary buffering
➤ Occurs in the proximal (PCT) and distal (DCT) convoluted tubules and collecting ducts.
➤ In the PCT, H^+ is secreted in exchange for Na^+, and combines with filtered HCO_3^- to form carbonic acid. This in turn dissociates into H_2O and CO_2 which moves freely into the tubular cell. There, the reaction is reversed and the HCO_3^- formed enters the interstitium and later the plasma. Thus, for every H^+ secreted, one HCO_3^- is reabsorbed.

➤ Some phosphate buffering takes place in the PCT, but most of it occurs in the DCT and collecting ducts.
➤ H^+ combines with secreted NH_3 to form NH_4^+, which is excreted in the urine.
➤ Ammonia buffering takes place mainly in the PCT and DCT.
➤ Buffering by bicarbonate results in bicarbonate reabsorption, whereas buffering with phosphate and ammonia results in bicarbonate regeneration.

How do you know the difference between 'open' and 'closed' buffer systems?
➤ **Closed buffers:** The total concentration of buffer within the cell is fixed, e.g. phosphate and haemoglobin. The addition of a strong acid or base results in maintenance of the pH, by shifting of the equation to the left or right, respectively. The buffering capacity is maximal when the pH = pKa of the buffer system, and is significantly reduced when the pH varies by more than 1 from the buffer's pKa.
➤ **Open buffers:** The total concentration of buffer within a compartment is not fixed, e.g. bicarbonate/carbonic acid system. One of the components (H_2CO_3) is fixed, while the other (HCO_3^-) varies inversely with the [H^+]. This is because CO_2 is highly permeable, therefore its intra– and extracellular concentrations are equal. As it is in equilibrium with H_2CO_3, it follows that the intracellular concentration of the latter is fixed. The buffering capacity increases as the concentration of the non-fixed component (HCO_3^-) and therefore intracellular pH increases, despite cell pH moving further away from the buffer's pKa.

How much acid is produced by the body per day?
The body produces metabolic and respiratory acids. Metabolic acids are produced from metabolism of amino acids, phoshoproteins and phospholipids, and amount to 70 μmol/min or 0.1 mol/day.
Respiratory acids are formed from CO_2 production and amount to 200 mL/min or 8 mmol/min which equals 12 mol/day.
Other sources of acid production include:
➤ lactic acid (strenuous exercise)
➤ ketoacids (diabetic ketoacidosis)
➤ failure of H^+ secretion by diseased kidneys (renal failure)
➤ ingestion of acidifying salts (NH_4Cl and $CaCl_2$).

What effects does chronic renal failure have on acid–base balance?
➤ More acid is produced by metabolism than is excreted. This depletes extracellular buffers and reduces plasma bicarbonate levels.
➤ Reduced total number of functioning nephrons → reduced production and secretion of ammonia → reduced buffering of urinary H^+ → reduced tubular secretion of H^+.
➤ Excess K^+ causes intracellular alkalosis, which inhibits H^+ secretion.
➤ Bicarbonate reabsorption and regeneration are reduced.
➤ Excess acid may be buffered by calcium carbonate in bone, so contributing to renal osteodystrophy.
➤ Haemoglobin levels are reduced due to depressed production of new red blood cells from a diminished erythropoietin secretion.
➤ Plasma proteins may be diminished in the presence of increased glomerular permeability in certain conditions (glomerulonephritis / nephrotic syndrome).

CHAPTER 26

Renal blood flow

The kidney receives 20–25% of cardiac output, i.e., 500–600 mL/min to each kidney.

More than 90% supplies the cortex via the renal artery, and less than 10% supplies the renal capsule and renal adipose tissue.

The cortex is supplied at 500 mL/min/100 g tissue. Some of this blood passes into the medulla, with perfusion rates of 100 mL/min/100 g tissue to the outer medulla and 20 mL/min/100 g tissue to the inner medulla.

HINT: REMEMBER THE RULE OF '5's

- 1/5 of cardiac output
- 500 mL/min to each kidney
- 500 mL/min/100 g tissue to the cortex
- 1/5 of this (100 mL/min/100 g tissue) to the outer medulla
- 1/5 of that (20 mL/min/100 g tissue) to the inner medulla

Describe the anatomy of the kidney

The renal artery enters each kidney at the hilum and divides into several branches. Interlobar arteries give rise to interlobular arteries which give rise to afferent arterioles, which supply the glomerular capillaries (site of filtration). Glomerular capillaries drain into efferent arterioles, which are portal vessels as they carry blood from one capillary network to another. In the outer two-thirds of the cortex, peritublar capillaries surround the proximal and distal convoluted tubules and collecting tubules. In the inner third of the cortex, the vasa recta surround the loops of Henle and collecting ducts.

What are the functions of renal blood flow?

- ➤ Provision of glucose and oxygen to meet the metabolic demands of renal tissue.
- ➤ Removal of CO_2 and other products of metabolism.
- ➤ Maintenance of GFR.
- ➤ Provision of O_2 for active reabsorption of sodium.

Describe the autoregulation of renal blood flow

Autoregulation describes the ability to maintain a constant renal blood flow (RBF) over a wide range of mean arterial pressures (MAP) or tissue perfusion pressures (PP) from 90–200 mmHg.

Myogenic theory – This is the most widely accepted explanation brought about by a direct contractile response of the afferent arteriolar smooth muscle to stretch. An increase in perfusion pressure results in smooth muscle contraction and an increase in the renal vascular resistance, so maintaining a constant blood flow.

Other factors affecting RBF include:

➤ Renal sympathetic nerve stimulation results in vasoconstriction of afferent arterioles thereby reducing RBF.

➤ Renal prostaglandins (PG) attenuate the SNS-induced vasoconstriction through vasodilation and thereby increasing RBF.

➤ Angiotensin 2 vasoconstricts the efferent arterioles more than the afferent arterioles, thus maintaining glomerular filtration rate (GFR).

➤ Tubuloglomerular feedback mechanism.

➤ Mediators present in blood vessel walls help to regulate GFR by vasodilatation (nitric oxide (NO)) or vasoconstriction (endothelin).

Describe the tubuloglomerular feedback (TGF)

This describes how the rate of flow through the tubules feeds back (negatively) to affect glomerular filtration. The mechanism has three components:

➤ **Sensor:** the macula densa in the distal tubular epithelium detecting fluid delivery within the tubule.

➤ **Transmission** of signal to the glomerulus.

➤ **Effector:** vascular smooth muscle in the afferent arteriole which adjusts GFR by vasodilatation or vasoconstriction.

Therefore, as the fluid load in the tubule increases, the afferent arteriole vasoconstricts and GFR is reduced. The converse is also true.

TGF is mediated by PG, thromboxane A2, NO and endothelin, and plays a role in RBF autoregulation.

How can renal blood flow be measured?

RBF can be calculated by plasma clearance of para-amino hippuric acid (PAH), as a modification of the Fick principle.

➤ **Fick principle:** Flow to an organ is equal to the uptake/excretion of a substance by an organ per unit time divided by the arteriovenous (A-V) concentration difference of that substance across that organ (L/min).

➤ **Plasma clearance:** the volume of plasma cleared of a substance per unit time (mL/min). PAH, an organic acid, is used because:

  ● It has a high extraction ratio (it is almost completely removed by the kidneys) via filtration and secretion, therefore its A-V concentration difference across the renal vascular bed is equal to the renal arteriolar concentration.

  ● It is neither utilised nor excreted by any other organ, therefore its peripheral venous plasma concentration is identical to its renal arterial concentration.

➤ Applying the Fick equation, PAH uptake by the kidney is given by the product of urine PAH concentration and urine flow. The A-V concentration difference is substituted by peripheral venous plasma concentration as explained above. This gives us the equation for clearance.

Clearance of PAH = Urine [PAH] × urine flow / plasma [PAH]

➤ Clearance helps us calculate renal plasma flow (RPF), since it is plasma and not blood which is filtered.

➤ RBF can then be deduced from RPF if the haematocrit (Hct) is known, by the equation: **RBF = RPF / 1-Hct**

What do you understand by the term glomerular filtration rate (GFR)?
This the volume of plasma filtered at the glomerulus per unit time.
  It is approximately 125 mL/min or 180 L/day.
  Values in women are ~10% lower than in men.

Filtration fraction is the ratio of GFR to RPF (~ 0.16–0.2).
RPF represents the total amount of potentially filterable fluid entering the kidneys (600–700 mL/min). Of this, 125 mL/min forms the GFR (20%) while the remainder continues into the efferent arterioles.

How can GFR be measured?
GFR can be calculated using the plasma clearance of a suitable substance (inulin/creatinine).

Clearance (GFR) = Urine concentration × Urine flow/ Plasma concentration

Ideally, the substance should have the following characteristics:
➤ freely filtered through the glomeruli (not bound to protein)
➤ not reabsorbed or secreted
➤ not metabolised
➤ not stored in the kidney
➤ no effect on the filtration rate
➤ not toxic
➤ easy to measure in plasma and urine.

Inulin, a polysaccharide with a molecular weight of 5200 Daltons meets all the criteria but, in practice, creatinine is used.
  GFR values calculated with either substance correspond quite well.
  Urine [creat] may be elevated due to tubular secretion, but this is cancelled out by plasma [creat], which is raised due to non-specific chromogens.

What factors affect GFR?
These are the same as those governing filtration across any capillary bed:
➤ permeability of capillaries
➤ size of capillary bed (surface area)
➤ hydrostatic and osmotic pressure gradients across the capillary wall (Starling's forces).

Capillary permeability
➤ Glomerular capillary wall is highly permeable due to its fenestrations.
➤ Neutral substances of < 4 nm diameter are freely filtered, but > 8 nm, their filtration approaches zero.
➤ Between 4 and 8 nm, their filtration is inversely proportional to diameter (Graham's law).
➤ The basement membrane's negative charge repels negatively charged ions, whose filtration is greatly reduced, e.g. albumin.
➤ The filtration of positively charged ions is slightly greater than that of neutral substances.

Size of capillary bed (surface area)
➤ Mesangial cells, located between the capillary endothelium and the basement membrane, have a contractile function, reducing the surface area available for filtration.
➤ Many vasoactive substances affect the mesangial cells, e.g. angiotensin 2 contracts while PGE2 relaxes.

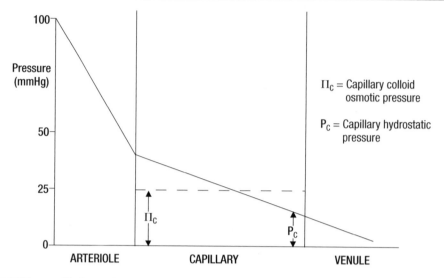

GRAPH 1.34 Hydrostatic and osmotic pressures within a typical vascular bed

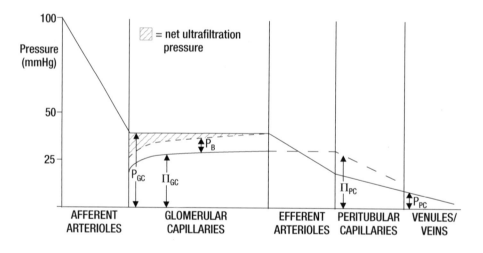

GRAPH 1.35 Hydrostatic and colloid osmotic pressures within the renal vascular bed

➤ **Starling's forces**
➤ The net filtration rate is a function of the forces favouring filtration and those opposing it, and can be described by the following equation:

$$\text{GFR} = K\!f\,[(P_{GC} - P_B) - (\Pi_{GC} - \Pi_B)]$$

Where:

$K\!f$ glomerular filtration coefficient (permeability × capillary bed surface area)
P_{GC} hydrostatic pressure in glomerular capillary
P_B hydrostatic pressure in Bowman's capsule
Π_{GC} colloid osmotic pressure in glomerular capillary
Π_B colloid osmotic pressure in Bowman's capsule

➤ P_{GC} is higher (45 mmHg) than in other capillary beds (32 mmHg) because:
  - afferent arterioles are short and straight
  - efferent arterioles have a relatively high resistance.
➤ P_{GC} favours filtration and is opposed by:
  - hydrostatic pressure in Bowman's capsule
  - osmotic pressure gradient across the glomerular capillaries ($\Pi_{GC} - \Pi_B$).
➤ Π_B is usually negligible and the osmotic pressure gradient is generally equal to the pressure exerted by the plasma proteins within the glomerular capillaries (Π_{GC}).
  The equation can therefore be expressed as:

$$GFR = Kf \; [P_{GC} - P_B - \Pi_{GC}]$$

➤ P_{GC} remains constant from afferent to efferent end of the glomerular capillary (45 mmHg), as does the P_B (10 mmHg).
➤ Π_{GC} rises from 20 mmHg at the afferent end to 35 mmHg at the efferent end because plasma proteins become progressively more concentrated as filtration occurs along the length of the capillaries.
➤ Just proximal to the efferent arteriole, the net ultrafiltration pressure is reduced to zero and filtration ceases.

TABLE 1.36 Starling pressures (mmHg) at the afferent and efferent arteriole

	Afferent end	Efferent end
P_{GC}	45	45
P_B	10	10
Π_{GC}	20	35
Net	15	0

CHAPTER 27

Renal handling of glucose, sodium and inulin

Using a straight line to represent the length of the proximal convoluted tubule (PCT), from the Bowman's capsule to the start of the loop of Henle, show the glucose, sodium and inulin concentrations. Explain the diagram and the physiology involved.

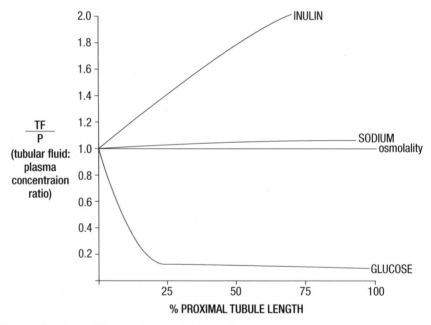

GRAPH 1.37 Renal handling of glucose, inulin and sodium

➤ In health, glucose is completely reabsorbed so its concentration falls to zero along the length of the PCT (sharp decline in the first part of the PCT, with slower decline further down).
➤ Sodium is almost completely reabsorbed and is followed by passive diffusion of water, so its concentration remains unchanged (straight line).
➤ Inulin is filtered but not reabsorbed, so its concentration rises (sloped positive curve).

TABLE 1.38 Renal handling of various substances in filtrate per 24 hours

Substance	Filtered	Reabsorbed	Secreted	Excreted	Percentage reabsorbed	Location*
Na^+ (meq)	26 000	25 850		150	99.4	P,L,D,C
K^+ (meq)	600	560	50	90	93.3	P,L,D,C
Urea (mmol)	870	460		410	53.0	P,L,D,C

Substance	Filtered	Reabsorbed	Secreted	Excreted	Percentage reabsorbed	Location*
Creatinine (mmol)	12	1	1	12		P,L,D,C
Glucose (mmol)	800	800			100.0	P
Water (mL)	180 000	179 000		1000	99.4	P,L,D,C

* P = proximal tubules; L = loops of Henle; D = distal tubules; C = collecting ducts.

What are the transport mechanisms involved?
➤ **Passive diffusion** down chemical or electrical gradients, e.g. sodium ions from tubular lumen into tubular cell.
➤ **Facilitated diffusion** down chemical or electrical gradients:
  ● co-transport (symport) of glucose, amino acids, bicarbonate and other electrolytes with sodium
  ● antiport mechanism involving Na^+ and H^+ across the tubule wall.
➤ **Active transport** against chemical or electrical gradients, e.g. movement of sodium from tubular cell into the interstitium via the Na^+-K^+-ATPase pump.

The driving force behind the reabsorption of sodium and other ions is the Na^+-K^+-ATPase pump, which acts at the basilar wall of the tubular cell. It extrudes 3 Na^+ into the interstitium in exchange for 2 K^+ that are pumped into the cell. This creates a Na^+ concentration gradient between the tubular lumen and cell, such that sodium diffuses readily into the cell from the lumen. The movement of other molecules and electrolytes is coupled to sodium reabsorption by antiport and symport mechanisms. Water diffuses along its concentration gradient. The K^+ that is pumped into the cell diffuses out into the interstitium along its concentration gradient.

How much glucose is filtered by the kidney, and how much can be reabsorbed?
➤ 100% of plasma glucose is filtered.
➤ Active transport mechanisms become saturated at higher concentrations of solute and their maximum rate of transport (reabsorption) is reached. This is known as the transport maximum (Tm) for a given solute.
➤ Glucose reabsorption is proportional to the amount filtered, and hence to the plasma concentration multiplied by the GFR up to the transport maximum, which is about 180 mg/dL or 10 mmol/L of venous plasma.
➤ Once the renal threshold for glucose is reached, not all the filtered glucose is reabsorbed and glucose starts to appear in the urine.

What physiological factors increase the GFR?
These are the same factors that govern filtration across any capillary bed:
➤ permeability of capillaries
➤ size of capillary bed (surface area)
➤ hydrostatic and osmotic pressure gradients across the capillary wall (Starling's forces).

The GFR is proportional to glomerular capillary pressure, which in turn depends on:
➤ local autoregulation, mediated by renal sympathetic nerves
➤ mean arterial pressure.

CHAPTER 28

Fluid compartments

Describe the major fluid components of the body in the adult

➤ **Total body water** (TBW) varies depending on age, size, gender and fat content. It is approximately 60% of body weight in the average adult male (i.e. 42 L) and 50% in the average adult female. The remainder of the weight is made up of protein, minerals and fat. The main components of TBW are the extracellular and intracellular compartments.

➤ **Intracellular fluid** (ICF) makes up two-thirds of TBW (i.e. 28 L).

➤ **Extracellular fluid** (ECF) makes up one-third of TBW (i.e. 14 L). This is divided into:
  - **interstitial fluid** (ISF), which makes up 75% of the ECF (i.e. 9.5 L)
  - **plasma**, making up 25% of the ECF (i.e. 3.5 L)
  - **transcellular fluids** (TCF) (i.e. 1 L), which are secreted fluids that are separated from the plasma by an epithelial layer (pleural, peritoneal, gastrointestinal fluids, CSF, intra-ocular fluids, sweat, saliva and bile).

➤ **Total blood volume** (TBV) consists of plasma and red cell volume, and is 5–6 L.

TABLE 1.39 Fluid compartments for a 70 kg male

Compartment	% BW	% TBW	% ECF	Volume (L)
TBW	~ 60			42
ICF	40	67		28
ECF	20	33		14
➤ ISF	15	10.5	75	9.5
➤ plasma	5	3.5	25	3.5
➤ TCF	< 1			1.0

Compare the adult with the neonate fluid compartments

TABLE 1.40 Comparison of neonatal and adult fluid compartments

Compartment	Adult	Neonate
TBW (% BW)	60	75–85
Fat (% BW)	20–25	5–15
ECF (% BW)	20	30–45
ICF (% BW)	40	< 40
Plasma (% BW)	5	5

Note that in premature babies, ECF exceeds ICF.

How are the body compartment volumes estimated?

Dilutional techniques are used to estimate compartment volumes. An indicator dye is injected into the compartment to be measured. The dye should distribute throughout that compartment, but remain contained within it. The concentration of the dye is measured and the mass administered is known. Thus, using the formula for volume of distribution (V_D = mass of dye/concentration), the compartment volume can be estimated.

Some compartments are derived (ICF, ISF and TBV).

TABLE 1.41 Methods of measurement of fluid compartments

Compartment	Characteristic of indicator	Indicator
TBW	Freely diffusible substance	Deuterium oxide
		Antipyrine
ECF	Substances that do not enter cells	Inulin
		Thiocyanate
		Thiosulphate
ICF		*TBW – ECF*
Plasma	Substances confined to plasma	Radiolabelled albumin
		Evan's blue dye
Red cell volume		Radiolabelled red cells
TBV		*Plasma volume × 100 / (100 – haematocrit)*
Interstitial fluid		*ECF – plasma volume*

What factors regulate body water?

Water balance governs the ICF and sodium balance regulates the ECF compartments.

The control of TBW is linked to the secretion of antidiuretic hormone (ADH, vasopressin) by the posterior pituitary.

ADH is secreted in response to:
➤ Hyperosmolarity (threshold 1–2%) detected by osmoreceptors in the hypothalamus, outside the blood brain barrier. Similarly, osmoreceptors stimulate thirst.
➤ Volume depletion (ECF) detected by low-pressure baroreceptors in great veins, atria and pulmonary vessels, and high pressure baroreceptors in the carotid sinus and aortic arch (threshold 7% change in volume).
➤ Angiotensin II (AGII).
➤ Other: pain, exercise, stress, emotion, nausea and vomiting, standing, nicotine, morphine, barbiturates, carbamazepine.

Its secretion is reduced in response to:
➤ low osmolarity
➤ increased ECF volume
➤ alcohol.

The renal effects of ADH on water balance include:
➤ increased water permeability in cortical collecting tubule (V2 receptors)
➤ increased water and urea permeability in medullary collecting tubule
➤ increased retention of water
➤ reduced urine volume.

Other ADH effects include:
➤ release of factor 8 by the endothelium (V2)
➤ platelet aggregation and degranulation (V1)
➤ arteriolar vasoconstriction (V1).

Sodium balance governs the ECF volume (as water passively diffuses across membranes when sodium is reabsorbed) and is regulated by:

➤ Dietary sodium intake.
➤ ECF volume (baroreceptors) and ADH secretion.
➤ GFR and tubuloglomerular feedback.
➤ Renin-angiotensin-aldosterone system:
  • efferent arteriolar vasoconstriction to maintain GFR
  • direct sodium reabsorption
  • secretion of aldosterone from adrenal cortex
  • increased ADH
  • increased thirst (water retention)
  • negative feedback on renin release.
➤ Aldosterone and other adrenocortical hormones:
  • reabsorption of NaCl (30–90 min latent period)
  • excretion of K^+
  • secretion of H^+
  • accompanied by changes in ADH.
➤ Rate of tubular secretion of K^+ and H^+.
➤ Atrial natriuretic peptide (ANP) and other natriuretic hormones:
  • secreted by atrial myocytes in response to atrial stretch due to ECF expansion (from high NaCl intake or IV infusion of saline)
  • actions include natriuresis (by an increase in GFR and tubular excretion of sodium), reduction in BP (by reduced responsiveness of vascular smooth muscle to vasoconstrictors), and reduced secretion of aldosterone, ADH, renin and consequently AGII.

What is the effect of a sudden IV infusion of 5% dextrose?
➤ 5% dextrose is a hypotonic solution and therefore gets distributed equally throughout all the fluid compartments. It can be thought of as water because the dextrose gets metabolised leaving behind water, which diffuses freely.
➤ Intravascular volume will thus increase only minimally (by approximately 70 mL if 1 L was administered).
➤ This is less than the 7–10% threshold needed to stimulate the baroreceptors.
➤ However, the plasma osmolarity will decrease enough to stimulate the osmoreceptors (1–2% threshold) and therefore ADH secretion will decrease, increasing renal water excretion.

What is the effect of an IV infusion of 1 L 0.9% saline solution?
➤ This is an isotonic solution.
➤ Sodium will diffuse from areas of high concentration to those of lower concentrations and will be followed by water.
➤ The cell membrane is impermeable to sodium and thus the distribution of the saline (water) administered will be confined to the ECF with 75% (750 mL) in the ISF and 25% (250 mL) in the plasma.
➤ The plasma expansion from 3.5 L to 3.75 L is enough (7% increase) to be detected by the baroreceptors and ADH secretion is reduced.
➤ The increased sodium load and ECF expansion will cause an increase in ANP secretion and natriuresis, and inhibition of the renin-angiotensin-aldosterone system.

CHAPTER 29

Osmoregulation

Define the following terms:

Osmosis: the diffusion of water molecules (solvent) across a semi-permeable membrane, from a dilute solution to a concentrated solution.

Osmotic pressure: the pressure required to prevent solvent migration by osmosis across a semi-permeable membrane. Applying pressure to the more concentrated solution can prevent the movement of water to the region of greater solute concentration.

Osmole: reflects the concentration of osmotically active particles in solution.
1 osmole = amount of solute that exerts an osmotic pressure of 1 atm when placed in 22.4 L of solution at 0°C.
For substances that do not dissociate, e.g. glucose, 1 osmole = 1 mole.
For substances that dissociate into two osmotically active particles, e.g. NaCl, 1 osmole = 1 mole/2 (i.e. 1 mole = 2 osmoles).

Osmolarity: the number of osmoles (or mosmoles) of solute in 1 L of solution, osm/L. As it is temperature-dependent, it poses a potential source of inaccuracy.

Osmolality: the number of osmoles (or mosmoles) in 1 kg of water (pure solvent), osm/kg. It is not influenced by temperature and is therefore more accurate than osmolarity.

How do you calculate plasma osmolality?
A simple formula, which sums up the major solutes, may be used:

$$(2 \times Na^+) + glucose + urea$$

This adds up to approximately 290 mosmol/kg H_2O.

What are the colligative properties of water?
These are properties of solutions that depend on the number of solute particles, but not on their nature, i.e. they depend on the osmolarity of a solution:
➤ lowering of vapour pressure
➤ elevation of boiling point
➤ depression of freezing point
➤ osmotic pressure.

How do you calculate osmotic pressure?
Dilute solutions behave in a similar way to ideal gases, i.e. osmotic pressure (P) is related to temperature (T) and volume (V) in the same way that an ideal gas is.

Applying the van't Hoff equation: **PV = nRT**

Where:

n = number of particles and **R** = universal gas constant (n/V = osmolality), we can calculate the value of osmotic pressure of plasma as follows:

$$P = nRT/V$$
$$= 290 \text{ mosm/kg } H_2O \times 8.32 \text{ J/K} \times 307 \text{ K}$$
$$= 740729.6 \text{ Pa}$$
$$= 740.7 \text{ kPa}$$
$$= 7.33 \text{ atm } (5629.3 \text{ mmHg})$$

How do you measure osmotic pressure?

Osmometers capable of detecting temperature changes of $0.002°C$ are used. They utilise one or more of the colligative properties of water:

➤ 1 mole of a solute added to 1 kg of water will depress the freezing point by $1.86°C$ (e.g. grit salt on the icy roads causes the ice to melt).

➤ The molar concentration of a solute causes a directly proportional reduction in vapour pressure (Raoult's law).

What is oncotic pressure (colloid osmotic pressure)?

Electrolytes account for more than 99% of plasma osmolality and osmotic pressure. Plasma proteins contribute to the remaining < 1%, which is the colloid osmotic (oncotic) pressure, and amounts to 25–28 mmHg. Despite its small number, oncotic pressure is significant, as it is the major determinant of retention of fluid within the capillaries.

What are the body's osmoreceptors?

These are cells of the anterior hypothalamus, located outside the blood brain barrier. They respond to changes in osmolality and stimulate thirst and the secretion of vasopressin.

What are the actions of vasopressin (antidiuretic hormone, ADH)?

ADH stimulates V2 receptors on collecting ducts which increases adenylate cyclase activity. This causes fusion of pre-formed water channels on the apical membrane resulting in increased permeability of the collecting ducts to water.

Other ADH effects include:

➤ stimulates thirst

➤ release of factor VIII by the endothelium

➤ platelet aggregation and degranulation

➤ arteriolar vasoconstriction

➤ glycogenolysis in the liver

➤ brain neurotransmitter

➤ secretion of ACTH from the anterior pituitary gland.

What stimulates water intake?

Multiple factors are involved in regulating water intake.

➤ An increase in plasma osmolality (with effective increase in osmotic pressure) stimulates osmoreceptors in the anterior hypothalamus, which in turn control thirst and simulate us to drink. ADH release also stimulates thirst.

➤ Extracellular fluid (ECF) volume depletion stimulates the renin-angiotensin system. The resultant increase in circulating angiotensin II acts on a specialised receptor in the diencephalon concerned with thirst. Baroreceptors appear to be involved as well when ECF volume is low.

➤ Dryness of the pharyngeal mucous membranes causes the sensation of thirst.

➤ Psychological and social factors also play a role.

CHAPTER 30

Action potentials

Questions about nerve action potentials (AP) are fairly common. Consider starting off by drawing a diagram of an AP. Remember to be accurate with the values of your membrane potentials.

Can you describe the action potential travelling along a mixed nerve?

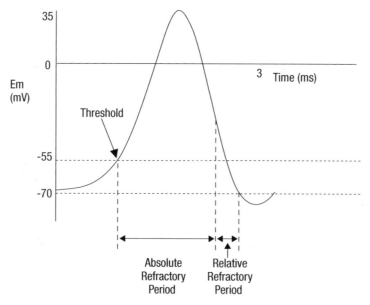

GRAPH 1.42 Mixed nerve action potential

The term action potential describes the depolarisation, above threshold potential, and subsequent repolarisation of a nerve axon resulting in the propagation of a nerve impulse along that axon. The easiest way to describe this is in a series of steps relating to the diagram of the AP:

➤ The inside of each cell in the body is negative relative to its surroundings. The potential difference across the cell membrane is called the membrane potential (E_m) and is governed by the membrane's relative permeability to sodium (Na^+) and potassium (K^+) ions. When the cell is at rest, it is relatively more permeable to K^+ than Na^+ and so the resting membrane potential approaches the equilibrium potential of K^+. In a mixed nerve this E_m is −70 mV.

➤ Nerve, muscle cells and pacemaker cells are able to generate APs. When a stimulus causes a movement of charge across the membrane there is a movement away from the resting membrane potential. If the inside of the cell becomes more positive, this is called depolarisation whereas becoming more negative is referred to as hyperpolarisation. Depolarisation in a nerve cell is caused by the movement of Na^+ ions into the cell.

➤ If a nerve cell becomes depolarised, e.g. by distortion opening Na^+ channels in the mechanoreceptors of the skin, the movement of the membrane potential towards zero causes opening of voltage-gated Na^+ channels. Once a Na^+ channel opens, it will close again automatically after a millisecond or so. Therefore, if the initial stimulus is not strong enough to cause enough Na^+ channels to open to allow enough Na^+ into the cell to bring the E_m to threshold potential, the membrane potential will fall away from zero and become more negative as the K^+ equilibrium is re-established. So, no AP will be generated.

➤ If, however, the initial stimulus is strong enough, enough channels will open to allow an influx of Na^+ that will raise the membrane potential to the threshold level of $-55\,mV$. If this level is reached, then a positive feedback effect occurs on the Na^+ channels causing large numbers of them to open. Consequently, there is an explosive influx of Na^+ raising the membrane potential above 0, to $+35\,mV$. So, the AP is an 'all-or-nothing' event – the membrane either reaches threshold level or it does not.

➤ These Na^+ channels opened by positive feedback will still close rapidly as before. As the membrane potential nears the equilibrium potential of Na^+ ($+70\,mV$), the diffusion of Na^+ ions into the cell slows. The maximum membrane potential is defined by the relationship of the Na^+/K^+ equilibrium and, therefore, the size of the AP is fixed, and not dependent on the size of the stimulus. Similarly, the duration is fixed, because this is dependent on the length of time that the Na^+ channels remain open, and this time is fixed.

➤ Once the Na^+ channels close, repolarisation occurs by the movement of K^+ ions out of the cell to restore the resting membrane potential. This happens as voltage gated K^+ channels open in the face of an AP, allowing the movement of the K^+ out of the cell along its diffusion gradient. These K^+ channels remain open after the Na^+ ones have closed, therefore allowing the resting membrane potential to be re-established. This process is called delayed rectification. Following only a few APs, the net change in number of Na^+ and K^+ ions in and outside the cell is small. However, after many APs, the changes become significant and the balance across the membrane is restored using the Na^+-K^+ pumps.

➤ An inactivated Na^+ channel cannot reopen until it has returned to near resting membrane potential. This explains the absolute refractory period that follows each AP, where the nerve cell cannot be excited, no matter how large the stimulus. The relative refractory period follows the absolute, and, here, another AP can be generated with a supra-maximal stimulus.

How does the AP move along the axon of a nerve?

In an unmyelinated axon the AP moves rather like a wave; local currents spreading in front of the AP cause a change in membrane potential and bring the membrane to threshold potential to spark the propagation of the AP. The AP can only flow in one direction as the axon behind it will be refractory.

Myelin acts as insulation because the charge cannot leak from the axon in an area covered by the myelin, and so charge density is maintained. In the 'nodes of Ranvier', i.e. the spaces between the myelinated areas, the charge can escape; the net effect is that the AP jumps from node to node. This is called saltatory conduction. So, the myelin increases the AP's velocity, and its insulating effect allows axons to be of smaller diameter (without myelination, conduction is fastest in axons with larger diameters).

What is the Gibbs-Donnan equilibrium?
> 'Diffusion of permeable ions across a semipermeable membrane down their concentration gradient is balanced by the electrostatic attraction of impermeable ions (e.g. proteins) trapped on the inside of the membrane.'

What is the Nernst equation?

The Nernst equation calculates the electrical potential for an individual ion, thus helping to predict how each ion affects the cell membrane potential. It represents the electrical potential required to balance a given ionic concentration gradient across a membrane so that there is no net flux.

$$E_m = \frac{RT}{ZF} \times \ln\frac{[ion]^{OUT}}{[ion]^{IN}}$$

Where:

E_m Membrane equilibrium potential
R   Universal gas constant
T   Absolute temperature
Z   Valency
F   Faraday's constant

Because R, T and F are constants and Z is one for the majority of ions that we are interested in, the Nernst equation can be simplified to:

$$E_m = 61.5 \times \log_{10}\frac{[ion]^{OUT}}{[ion]^{IN}}$$

What is the Goldman constant field equation?

This calculates the value of the overall membrane potential taking into account the permeabilities and concentration gradients of each ion.

$$V = \frac{RT}{ZF} \times \ln\frac{P[Na]^{OUT}}{P[Na]^{IN}} + \frac{P[K]^{OUT}}{P[K]^{IN}} + \frac{P[Cl]^{IN}}{P[Cl]^{OUT}}$$

CHAPTER 31

Cerebral blood flow

Cerebral function is dependent upon cerebral blood flow (CBF) and oxygenation. An understanding of the physiology of cerebral blood flow regulation is essential in order to manage patients who may have decompensated intracranial pathology or injuries.

Basic concepts
➤ Global CBF: 50 mL/100 g brain tissue/minute.
➤ White matter: 20 mL/100 g/min.
➤ Grey matter: 70 mL/100 g/min.
➤ Resting oxygen consumption of the brain: 50 mL/min (20% of total body oxygen requirements).
➤ Regional CBF varies depending on metabolic rates of local areas of brain.
➤ CBF exhibits autoregulation – the maintenance of constant blood flow despite changes in cerebral perfusion pressure (CPP).
➤ CPP = mean arterial pressure (MAP) – [Intracranial Pressure (ICP) + CVP]
   Normal CPP is approximately 80 mmHg.

Cerebral blood flow – myogenic theory vs. local metabolites
CBF is autoregulated between a MAP range of 50 to 150 mmHg (curve is shifted to the right in hypertensive patients).

Myogenic theory of cerebral autoregulation
A change in perfusion pressure results in a myogenic response in the cerebral vascular smooth muscle in order to maintain constant cerebral blood flow. For example, a hypertensive response during exercise with an increase in MAP results in cerebral vasoconstriction thus keeping CBF constant. Conversely, a fall in MAP will result in cerebral vascular smooth muscle relaxation causing vasodilatation thus maintaining CBF.

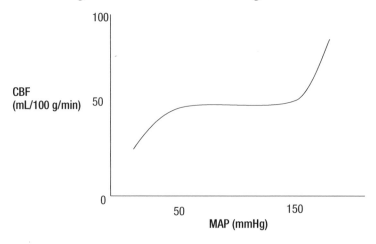

GRAPH 1.43 Autoregulation of cerebral blood flow

Metabolic theory of cerebral blood flow

CBF and cerebral metabolism are coupled. Thus, regional CBF varies with metabolic activity. Products of metabolism (H^+/K^+/adenosine/nitric oxide) cause vasodilatation. Thus, CBF matches metabolic requirements.

What are the effects of changes in PaO_2 and $PaCO_2$ on CBF?

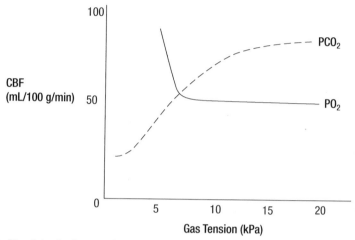

GRAPH 1.44 Physiological control of cerebral blood flow

➤ CBF increases linearly between a $PaCO_2$ range of 3 kPa to 10 kPa. Outside this range CO_2 reactivity is lost. Clinical implication – hypocapnia can result in intense cerebral vasoconstriction and ischaemia, hypercapnia can result in increased intracranial blood volume, which may result in a rise in ICP.
➤ CBF increases below a PaO_2 of 8 kPa due to hypoxic vasodilatation. Clinical implication: in patients with head injuries hypoxia may lead to further rises in ICP and result in brain ischaemia.

Do anaesthetic drugs have any effect on CBF?
➤ **Volatiles:** all increase CBF and reduce $CMRO_2$ thus uncoupling CBF from $CMRO_2$.
➤ **N_2O:** increases CBF and increases $CMRO_2$.
➤ **NMBA:** do not affect CBF.
➤ **Induction drugs:** With the exception of ketamine, all other induction agents reduce $CMRO_2$, CBF and ICP. Ketamine increases ICP.

How does temperature affect CBF?
Cerebral metabolic requirement for oxygen ($CMRO_2$) falls by 7% per 1°C fall in core body temperature. As a result, CBF parallels this reduction in $CMRO_2$.

What effect does brain injury have on cerebral blood flow?
Brain injury can lead to loss of cerebral autoregulation in injury-affected areas of the brain, resulting in the development of a pressure-dependent perfusion area. Thus, a fall in CPP may lead to secondary ischaemic brain injury.

What is the Monro-Kellie doctrine?
The skull is a rigid box containing brain tissue (80%), blood (12%) and CSF (8%). The volume of the box is constant, so an increase in volume of any one of the intracranial con-

stituents must be accompanied by a parallel reduction in the volume of another constituent if intracranial pressure (ICP) is to remain constant.

What is the normal ICP?
➤ 10–15 mmHg – normal.
➤ Above 20 mmHg – elevated ICP.

What are the common causes of raised ICP?
➤ **CSF** – hydrocephalus.
➤ **Brain** – tumours/oedema/contusions.
➤ **Blood** – haematoma/cerebral aneurysm.

Draw a graph to show how ICP is related to intracranial volume (ICV)

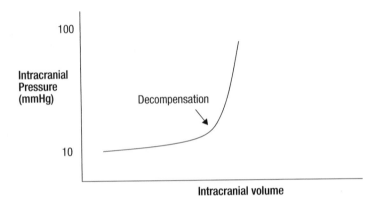

GRAPH 1.45 Effect of intracranial volume on intracranial pressure

As intracranial volume increases (e.g. cerebral oedema secondary to a traumatic brain injury) there is initially no rise in ICP as compensatory mechanisms occur such as a reduction in intracranial venous blood volume and an increase in CSF absorption combined with CSF movement into the spinal compartment. When these mechanisms are exhausted any further small increase in intracranial volume results in a large increase in ICP – i.e. decompensation has occurred.

What is the vasodilatory cascade?
In head-injured patients, the vasodilatory cascade describes the viscious cycle that develops if there is a reduction in cerebral perfusion pressure. Conversely, the vasoconstriction cascade describes the treatment of the above situation.

Vasodilatory cascade:

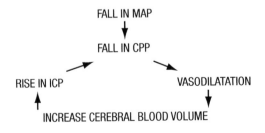

Vasoconstriction cascade:

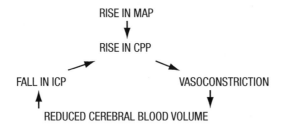

Describe the physiological management of the head-injured patient

Applying the above physiological principles, the following goals are aimed for when managing patients with head injuries:

➤ **ABC** approach.
➤ **Maintain oxygenation** ($PaO_2 > 10\,kPa$) – hypoxia will cause cellular ischaemia and raise ICP through vasodilatation.
➤ **Maintain CPP** (> 80 mmHg) – to ensure adequate cerebral blood flow and to prevent the vasodilatory cascade. May require fluids +/– vasopressors. ICP should ideally be monitored. Ensure good venous drainage of the head: 30° head up tilt, do not obstruct venous drainage with endotracheal tube ties – use tape.
➤ **Reduce ICP** – maintain normocapnia – prevent hypercapnia and hypoxia, both of which will increase cerebral blood volume. Consider use of furosemide (0.25–1.0 mg/kg)/mannitol (0.25–1.0 g/kg) or hypertonic saline.
➤ **Reduce CMRO$_2$** – consider infusions of propofol or midazolam or in certain situations thiopentone. Treat pyrexia. Therapeutic hypothermia is not proven to be of benefit in head-injured patients.
➤ **Prevent/treat seizures** – which causes a dramatic increase in CMRO$_2$.
➤ Maintain **normoglycaemia**.
➤ Do not administer hypotonic fluids such as 5% dextrose which will increase brain oedema.

CHAPTER 32

Cerebrospinal fluid

Cerebrospinal fluid (CSF) is the clear colourless fluid that bathes the brain and spinal cord acting as a fluid layer for protection of the central nervous system (CNS).

Where is CSF produced?
➤ CSF is produced by the choroid plexuses located in the third, fourth and lateral ventricles.
➤ Produced at a rate of approximately 0.3 mL per minute.
➤ Total volume of CSF is approximately 150 mL, which equates to 10% of intracranial volume.
➤ 450 mL of CSF is produced per day and so CSF volume is replaced three times per 24 hours.
➤ CSF is derived from plasma filtration and subsequent secretion by the choroid plexuses.
➤ CSF is one of the three determinants of intracranial pressure (the other two being brain tissue and blood volume).
➤ In situations of raised intracranial pressure CSF production remains relatively constant, however, CSF absorption increases thereby reducing total CSF volume as a compensatory mechanism.

Describe the circulation of CSF
➤ CSF flows from the lateral ventricles through the foramen of Monro into the third ventricle and from there via the aqueduct of Sylvius into the fourth ventricle.
➤ CSF leaves the ventricular system via the midline foramen of Magendie and lateral foramen of Lushka, entering the subarachnoid space of the brain and spinal cord.
➤ CSF is absorbed into the dural venous sinuses via arachnoid villi and granulations that project into the dural sinuses.

What is the relevance of the blood brain barrier (BBB)?
➤ Plasma constituents do not pass freely into the CSF and this phenomenon is the BBB.
➤ Anatomical and physiological factors involved in maintaining the BBB are:
  • tight junctions and fenestrated choroidal capillaries within the brain
  • specialised bidirectional transport system for ions, glucose and amino-acids.

Describe the normal CSF composition
Reference values for CSF are as follows:

Protein	0.15–0.45 g/L
Osmolality	280–300 mmol/L
Sodium	135–145 mmol/L
Potassium	2.6–3.0 mmol/L
Chloride	115–125 mmol/L
Calcium	1.00–1.40 mmol/L
Magnesium	1.2–1.5 mmol/L
Lactate	1.1–2.4 mmol/L
pH	7.28–7.40
Creatinine	50–110 umol/L
Glucose	2.8–4.4 mmol/L
Urea	3.0–6.5 mmol/L

A comparison of the composition of CSF and plasma reveals that:
➤ CSF proteins are ~1% that of plasma, resulting in reduced buffering capability
➤ CSF calcium levels are ~50% that of plasma
➤ CSF glucose levels are ~60% that of plasma
➤ CSF chloride and magnesium levels are higher than plasma.

What investigations may be performed on a CSF sample?
Important information on CSF can be derived from the following parameters.
➤ Opening pressure – elevated in raised intracranial pressure.
➤ Macroscopic appearance, e.g. xanthochromia.
➤ Total and differential cell count.
➤ Bacterial culture and sensitivity.
➤ Protein and glucose.
➤ Analysis of immunoglobulins (detect chronic CNS inflammatory conditions).
➤ Cytology.

What changes in CSF cell counts occur with CNS infection?
CSF normally contains a small number of cells (usually lymphocytes and monocytes) and the total cell count is less than 5 cells/mm³. An increase in cell counts suggests either an infection of the CNS, or a number of CNS pathological conditions. The differential cell count provides further information regarding the possible cause of the CNS disease.
➤ **Increased neutrophils** may indicate bacterial meningitis. Other causes of an increased neutrophil count include a cerebral abscess, following seizures and following CNS hemorrhage.
➤ **Increased lymphocytes** may indicate viral meningitis. Lymphocyte counts are also elevated in meningitis due to TB, syphilis, fungal and parasitic infections. Degenerative diseases of the CNS, such as multiple sclerosis, will also generate elevated lymphocyte counts.
➤ **'Mixed reaction'**, an increase in neutrophils, lymphocytes and plasma cells. This is characteristic of TB meningitis, fungal meningitis and chronic bacterial meningitis.
➤ **Increased plasma cells** is a feature of TB meningitis.
➤ **Leukaemic cells** indicates meningeal infiltration by haematological malignancy.

Can biochemical analysis of CSF be diagnostic?

➤ **CSF total protein:** The CSF normally contains less than 0.45 g/L protein. Increased levels may be found in:
  - infection
  - blood contamination
  - chronic inflammatory disorders of the CNS (TB, syphilis, Guillain-Barré).

➤ **CSF electrophoresis:** Electrophoretic separation of CSF proteins and detection of CSF immunoglobulin.

  CSF immunoglobulin can arise from three causes:
  1 secondary to an increase in plasma immunoglobulin, e.g. multiple myeloma
  2 impairment of the blood brain barrier
  3 local synthesis in the CNS, e.g. in multiple sclerosis the increase in CSF immunoglobulin is characterised by an oligoclonal pattern of immunoglobulin synthesis and this can be detected in 90% of patients with MS.

➤ **CSF glucose:** Low levels of CSF glucose suggest:
  - infection (local metabolism by white cells)
  - hypoglycemia (although CSF glucose is of limited diagnostic utility and the plasma glucose concentration must be known in order to interpret the CSF glucose level properly).

➤ **Polymerase chain reaction (PCR)** is a technique to rapidly amplify a defined region of DNA or RNA. PCR has been used to detect the presence of bacterial pathogens (e.g. syphilis and TB) and viral pathogens (e.g. HIV) in the CSF.

CHAPTER 33

Autonomic nervous system

Many anaesthetic agents and neuroaxial blocks interfere with the autonomic nervous system. However, there are occasions when we seek to manipulate the autonomic system deliberately, using various drugs (e.g. inotropes, β-blockers) and manoeuvres (e.g. valsalva). This question has a wide scope and can lead onto a variety of topics including the vagus nerve, autonomic reflexes and drugs acting on the autonomic system.

What is the autonomic nervous system?
The autonomic nervous system (ANS) is a collection of nerves and ganglia that are involved in the involuntary control of homeostasis and the stress response.

Describe the structure of the autonomic nervous system
➤ The ANS consists of two divisions, the parasympathetic nervous system (PNS) and the sympathetic nervous system (SNS). The PNS is involved in 'Rest and Digest' processes (picture Mr Parasympathetic sitting on the toilet, sphincters open and reading a newspaper with eyes accommodated). The SNS is involved in 'Fight or Flight' processes (just imagine what you are going to feel like at the exam – dilated pupils, sweaty, tachycardic, tachypnoeic, dry mouth and shivering!).
➤ The ANS receives afferent information from chemoreceptors, baroreceptors, mechanoreceptors and from regions within the central nervous system. Once processed, it relays this information through efferent pathways to target tissues (e.g. cardiac muscle, smooth muscle and glands).
➤ The efferent pathways of the PNS and SNS consist of a pre-ganglionic fibre, an autonomic ganglion and a post-ganglionic fibre. (N.B. the exception to this is the SNS innervation of the adrenal gland where there is only a single pre-ganglionic fibre that terminates on the adrenal medulla. The adrenal medulla then acts like a glorified 'post-ganglionic' fibre and releases neurotransmitters/hormones into the bloodstream).

Pre-ganglionic fibres (myelinated type B fibres):
➤ The cell bodies of the PNS pre-ganglionic fibres lie within the nuclei of III, VII, IX and X cranial nerves and also in the lateral grey horns of the second to fourth sacral segments. These fibres are long and form the craniosacral outflow tract.
➤ The cell bodies of the SNS pre-ganglionic fibres lie within the lateral grey horns of the first to twelfth thoracic segments and the first to third lumbar segments. These fibres are short and form the thoraco-lumbar outflow tract.

Autonomic ganglia:
➤ The PNS ganglia are known as terminal ganglia as they are located close to or within the wall of the target tissue.
➤ The SNS consists of two types of ganglia: the paravertebral ganglia (also called the sympathetic trunk) and the prevertebral ganglia. The paravertebral ganglia lie on either side of the vertebral column from the base of the skull to the coccyx. The prevertebral

ganglia (e.g. coeliac, superior mesenteric and inferior mesenteric ganglia) lie anterior to the vertebral column next to the major arteries.
➤ White rami communicantes connect SNS pre-ganglionic fibres to paravertebral ganglia.

Post-ganglionic fibres (unmyelinated type C fibres):
➤ PNS post-ganglionic fibres are short and their cell bodies lie within the autonomic ganglia.
➤ SNS post-ganglionic fibres are long and their cell bodies lie within the autonomic ganglia.
➤ Grey rami communicantes connect SNS ganglia to spinal nerves.

Neurotransmitters:
➤ All PNS and SNS pre-ganglion fibres are cholinergic (they release acetylcholine).
➤ Whereas all PNS post-ganglionic fibres are also cholinergic, only those SNS post-ganglionic fibres innervating sweat glands are cholinergic.
➤ All other SNS post-ganglionic fibres are adrenergic (they release noradrenaline).
➤ The adrenal medulla which acts like a 'glorified' SNS post-ganglionic fibre releases adrenaline (80%) and noradrenaline (20%).

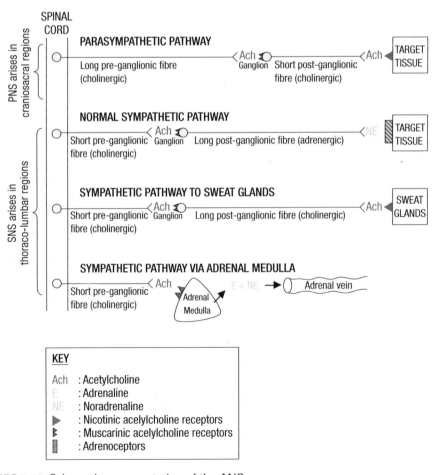

FIGURE 1.46 Schematic representation of the ANS

Receptors:

➤ Receptors sited within all autonomic ganglia and on the adrenal medulla are nicotinic acetylcholine receptors (nAChR).

➤ Receptors on the effector organs innervated by the PNS are muscarinic acetylcholine receptors (mAChR) while those innervated by the SNS are adrenergic receptors (either α or β).

➤ Muscarinic acetylcholine receptors are also located on sweat glands which are innervated by the SNS.

Which organs are not under dual innervation from the ANS?

Most target tissues receive dual innervation from the ANS. However, structures that only receive SNS innervation are the sweat glands, arrector pili muscles, adipose cells, kidneys and most blood vessels. The lacrimal glands only receive PNS innervation.

Compare and contrast the PNS and SNS

TABLE 1.47 Comparison of the PNS and SNS

Function	Rest and Digest	Fight or Flight
Pre-ganglionic fibres	Craniosacral tract	Thoraco-lumbar tract
	Long	Short
	Cholinergic	Cholinergic
Ganglia	Terminal	Paravertebral or prevertebral
	nAChR	nAChR
Post-ganglionic fibres	Short	Long
	Cholinergic	Adrenergic
Target tissues	Dual innervation to most target tissues except lacrimal glands	Dual innervation to most target tissue except sweat glands, arrector pili muscles, adipose cells, kidneys, and most blood vessels
	mAChR	α and β receptors

CHAPTER 34

Child versus adult

Describe the physiological and anatomical differences between a neonate and an adult
This is a relatively straightforward question, but to answer it well you must structure your
answer as there is a considerable amount of information to get across in a short space of
time. Be systematic.

In comparison to adults, children differ in the following anatomical and physiological
ways.

Respiratory system:
- Relatively larger head, short neck, large tongue and narrow nasal passages.
- High anterior larynx (level C2/3 compared to C5/6 in the adult).
- Large U-shaped floppy epiglottis.
- Narrowest point of the larynx is at the level of the cricoid cartilage (in adults it is at the laryngeal inlet).
- Equal angles of mainstem bronchi.
- Obligate nasal breathers.
- Compliant chest wall with horizontal ribs.
- Diaphragmatic breathing > intercostal breathing.
- Diaphragm movement restricted by relatively large liver.
- Relatively fixed tidal volume. Increase in minute ventilation achieved by increasing respiratory rate.
- Higher alveolar ventilation 100–150 mL/kg/min compared with 60 mL/kg/min in adult.
- Lower FRC. FRC encroaches on closing volume until age 5, resulting in airway closure at end-expiration.
- Sinusoidal respiratory pattern, no end-expiratory pause (inspiratory:expiratory ratio 1:1).
- Higher basal oxygen consumption 6 mL/kg/min compared with 3.5 mL/kg/min in the adult.
- Higher risk of apnoea.
- As a result of all of the above points, hypoxaemia occurs more rapidly.

Cardiovascular system:
- Circulating blood volume 85 mL/kg compared with 70 mL/kg in adult.
- Neonatal myocardium consists of more non-contractile connective tissue.
- Stroke volume is relatively fixed.
- Cardiac output is therefore largely rate dependent and neonates tolerate bradycardia poorly.
- Cardiac output 200 mL/kg/min.
- Better developed parasympathetic system than sympathetic, meaning bradycardia occurs frequently with hypoxia or vagal stimulation.

➤ Asystole is the most common form of cardiac arrest and ventricular fibrillation is uncommon.
➤ Transitional circulation may revert to fetal circulation if neonate becomes hypoxic, acidotic, hypercapnic or hypothermic.
➤ Haemoglobin higher in neonate: 16–20 g/dL.
➤ Right ventricular mass equal to left ventricular mass until 6 months of age resulting in right axis deviation on the ECG.

Central nervous system:
➤ Myelination is incomplete in the first year of life.
➤ Skull non-rigid with open fontanelles.
➤ MAC infant > neonate > adult.
➤ More sensitive to opiate-induced respiratory depression and apnoea.
➤ Immature neuromuscular junction which is very sensitive to non-depolarising muscle relaxants but relatively resistant to suxamethonium (use 1.5 mg/kg).
➤ Spinal cord ends at L3 (L1 by age 2 years).

Renal system:
➤ Higher total body water (80%) at birth.
➤ Increased extracelluar fluid (ECF) resulting in higher volumes of distribution of drugs.
➤ Renal immaturity resulting in poor handling of water excess or excess sodium.
➤ Poor renal hydrogen ion excretion.
➤ Glucose reabsorption is limited.
➤ Glomerular filtration and tubular reabsorption reduced until 6 to 8 months of age.
➤ Renal blood flow is 6% of cardiac output at birth rising to 18% of cardiac output at 1 month (compared with 20% in adult).
➤ GFR at term is 30 mL/min increasing to 110 mL/min by age 2 years.

Liver:
➤ Immature liver has fewer selective pathways to metabolise drugs.
➤ Low hepatic glycogen stores means hypoglycaemia occurs readily with prolonged fasting.

Temperature homeostasis:
➤ Poor temperature regulation in neonates.
➤ Large body surface area to volume ratio.
➤ High heat loss.
➤ Higher thermoneutral temperature (temperature below which an individual is unable to maintain core body temperature) 32°C for a term infant compared with 28°C for an adult.
➤ Infants < 3 months of age cannot shiver.
➤ Utilise non-shivering brown fat thermogenesis.

CHAPTER 35

Pregnancy

Can you describe the physiological changes associated with pregnancy?

This question is best answered by considering each system in turn. The list below is not exhaustive, but should certainly be enough to pass.

Haematology:
➤ **Plasma volume increases:** this increases preload and V_D of polar drugs. It increases by 50% by term.
➤ **RBC mass increases:** but plasma increases more than RBC, causing physiological anaemia.
➤ **WBC increase:** to 12×10^9/L by term with a further increase to 30×10^9/L during labour.
➤ **Platelets reduce:** due to consumption.
➤ **Albumin decreases:** this increases the free active proportion of plasma-bound drugs.
➤ **Plasma oncotic pressure reduces:** increases the risk of oedema.
➤ **Plasma cholinesterase reduces:** the effect of suxamethonium is offset by the increased V_D.
➤ **Hypercoaguable:** all clotting factors increase except XI and XIII. BT, PT and APTT shortened. High risk of thromboembolic complications.
➤ **CRP and ESR increase.**

Cardiovascular system:
➤ **Stroke volume and heart rate increase:** cardiac output increases by up to 60% by term (8 L/min).
➤ **Systemic vascular resistance reduces:** reduction in DBP > SBP leading to an increased PP. This is due to oestrogen and progesterone. Maintenance of SVR is governed by sympathetic drive, which is diminished by central neuro-axial blockade.
➤ **Left ventricular mass increases:** ECG shows left axis deviation, ST depression and even a flat or inverted T-wave. Systolic murmur almost universal at term but note that a diastolic murmur is not normal.
➤ **Vena caval compression:** reduces venous return and preload, decreased cardiac output, decreased BP and engorged verterbral veins.
➤ **Aortic compression:** occurs from 20 weeks gestation. Increases afterload, decreases cardiac output and utero-placental blood flow. This is decreased by avoiding supine position and using at least 15° lateral tilt.

Respiratory system:
➤ **Anatomy:** capillary enlargement and mucosal congestion can lead to voice changes and difficulty breathing in some women. The diaphragm is elevated by 4 cm, thoracic circumference increases as the ribs 'splay' out and breathing becomes largely diaphragmatic by term.
➤ **Volumes:** FRC reduces by up to 20% and closing volume encroaches on FRC leading

to airway closure and increasing the risk of hypoxia. This is made worse when supine, obese or multiple pregnancy. V_T increases but TLC and VC remains unchanged.
- **Ventilation:** respiratory rate and minute ventilation increase. Dead space increases due to bronchodilation.
- **Mechanics:** chest wall compliance reduces but lung compliance remains unchanged.
- **Oxygen consumption increases:** by up to 60%, increasing the risk of developing hypoxia during induction of anaesthesia.
- **ABG:** pH increases (to ~7.5), PO_2 increases (to ~14 kPa), PCO_2 reduces due to hyperventilation (to ~3.5 kPa) and HCO_3^- reduces (to ~18 mmol/L).

Gastrointestinal system:
- **Barrier pressure reduces:** due to increased intragastric pressure.
- **Gastric emptying is reduced:** this occurs during labour due to the effects of pain and opiates.
- **Risk of aspiration increases:** this returns to normal levels 48 hours post partum.

Renal:
- **Renal blood flow and GFR increase:** by up to 50%. Urea and creatinine levels reduce.
- **Glycosuria and proteinuria:** common.

Central nervous system:
- **Epidural space reduces:** due to the engorged extradural venous plexus. CSF volume is also reduced. Hence reduced volumes of local anaesthetic agents are required during central neuroaxial blockade (reduce dose by one-third). There is also an increased risk of inadvertent intravascular catheter placement.
- **Anaesthesia:** MAC decreased. Inhalational induction faster (as raised MV more significant factor that raised CO in this case). Following labour, woman has reduced strength in respiratory muscles for around 4 hours. Anaesthesia compounds this effect and reduces ability to cough.

Endocrine:
- **Thyroid:** increases in T3 and T4, may suppress TSH.
- **Insulin:** increased secretion from hypertrophied beta cells, but increased production of 'anti-insulin' hormones, e.g. cortisol. Gestational diabetes can result. Glucose crosses placenta by facilitated diffusion to protect fetus from fluctuating maternal levels.

CHAPTER 36

Placental transfer

What are the main functions of the placenta?
➤ Gas exchange.
➤ Nutrient and waste exchange.
➤ Transfer of immune complexes.
➤ Hormone synthesis.

Describe the mechanisms by which substances are transferred across the placenta
Placental transfer is subject to exactly the same rules governing transfer of substances across all semi-permeable phospholipid membranes. Mechanisms of transfer include:
➤ **simple diffusion**, e.g. O_2 and CO_2
➤ **facilitated transport**, e.g. glucose
➤ **secondary active transport**, e.g. amino acids, with sodium being the primary substance for transport
➤ **active transport**, e.g. iron and calcium
➤ **pinocytosis**, e.g. IgG
➤ **bulk transport**.

What factors affect the transfer of substances across the placenta?
All substances present in the maternal circulation are potentially available to the fetus. The following factors govern transfer across the placenta.
➤ **Lipid solubility:** The more lipid-soluble something is, the more readily it will diffuse across a lipid membrane, and so the placenta.
➤ **Degree of ionisation:** The more ionised a substance is, the less easily it diffuses across the placenta.
➤ **Degree of protein binding:** Only the unbound ('free') substance is available to cross any membrane, and so a highly bound substance will not cross the placenta readily. Pregnant women have relatively lower total protein contents of their blood and so theoretically a higher free fraction of a given substance might be present.
➤ **pH:** This affects the degree of ionisation of the drug, as dictated by its pKa. Also, acidosis decreases protein binding.
➤ **Molecular weight:** If less than 600 Daltons, cross readily.
➤ **Concentration gradient across the placenta:** This affects speed of transfer.

Local anaesthetics are often used during labour. Describe the transfer of local anaesthetics from the mother to the fetus
➤ Bupivacaine is the most commonly used local anaesthetic, given either as epidural or subarachnoid injection. It is used because it has fewer motor effects than other drugs available and has a relatively long duration of action.
➤ It can cross the placenta, but less readily than lignocaine because its pKa is higher than lignocaine's and so it is more ionised at physiological pH.
➤ The fetus has a lower pH than its mother, and so there is a risk of 'ion trapping', where

the drug crosses into the fetus, becomes more ionised, and therefore cannot move out again. This effect is exacerbated if the fetus becomes more acidotic, risking local anaesthetic toxicity.

Describe the transfer of pethidine

➤ Pethidine is the most commonly used opioid for labour pain and can be prescribed by the midwives in most UK maternity units.
➤ It is a highly lipid-soluble drug and so it passes freely across the placenta reaching equilibrium in about 6 minutes and reaching maximum levels in the fetus at around 2–3 hours.
➤ It is metabolised to norpethidine, which is less lipid-soluble and therefore remains in the fetus much longer.
➤ Norpethidine has little analgesic value and causes sedation, respiratory depression and is pro-convulsant. Its half-life in the mother is up to around 20 hours, but in the neonate can be as much as 62 hours.

Describe the Bohr effect in relation to placental gas exchange

Consider drawing the oxyhaemoglobin dissociation curve and using it to illustrate your answer.

➤ The Bohr effect describes the movement to the left or right of the oxyhaemoglobin dissociation curve, depending on the surrounding CO_2 tension and so the pH.
➤ Ambient CO_2 diffuses into red blood cells and dissociates to form $H^+ + HCO_3^-$. This causes the curve to shift to the right, as there is a reduction in the affinity of haemoglobin for oxygen. This encourages offloading of oxygen to the tissues.
➤ This mechanism is important in the utero-placental circulation. As the mother's blood flows through the uterus it is exposed to the high CO_2 tensions generated by the fetus excreting CO_2. The CO_2 diffuses into the mother's red blood cells and dissociates as we have described. As the fetus offloads its CO_2 to its mother, who 'accepts' it, the fetus' curve moves left, while the maternal one moves right. This is called the 'double Bohr effect'.
➤ The fetal haemoglobin has a P_{50} of ~2.5 kPa and so lies to the left of the mother's whose P_{50} is ~3.5 kPa. This supports uptake of oxygen by the fetus.

How is the Haldane effect relevant to the placenta?

The Haldane effect describes the increased affinity of deoxygenated haemoglobin for CO_2 and vice versa. This is relevant across the placenta because as the fetus gives up CO_2 it increases its affinity for O_2, and as the mother gives up her O_2 her haemoglobin has an increased affinity for the CO_2. This is called the 'double Haldane effect'.

Describe the placental handling of the following anaesthetic drugs

➤ **Thiopentone:** Crosses the placenta rapidly but the neonate does not suffer excessive sedation unless doses exceed 8 mg/kg.
➤ **Suxamethonium:** Does not cross the placenta in significant quantities unless the mother suffers from pseudocholinesterase deficiency, allowing significant concentrations to be present in her blood for a prolonged amount of time. The normally decreased levels of pseudocholinesterase found in pregnancy are not clinically significant.
➤ **Non-depolarising neuromuscular blockers:** These fully ionised, bulky, poorly lipid-soluble drugs do not cross the placenta.
➤ **Ephedrine:** Crosses easily.

CHAPTER 37

Ageing

How does ageing alter physiology and how does this impact on your anaesthetic practice?

Approach this question using a systems-based technique. Remember that each elderly patient presenting for surgery is an amalgam of the presenting acute disease, the process of ageing and residual effects of any previous illness.

Ageing is an irreversible process, which causes gradual reduction in the reserve of each system. The process affects everyone at different speeds, and often the decline is not obvious until almost total loss of reserve occurs. It is important to make a global assessment addressing physical, psychological and relevant social issues.

Cardiovascular system:
➤ Fewer pacemaker cells, making atrial fibrillation and other arrhythmias increasingly common with age. A pre-operative ECG is essential to look for any underlying pathology. The tendency towards bradycardia (sinus or otherwise) is exaggerated during general anaesthesia, so consider the use of anticholinergic agents such as glycopyrollate.
➤ The compliance of the whole vascular system reduces. There is reduced compliance of the left ventricle, which hypertrophies in the face of increased afterload. Atherosclerosis is often present and contributes to the development of hypertension.
➤ Baroreceptor reflexes become less efficient with age and so compensation for a change in posture, for example, is reduced, which can lead to hypotension. The tachycardic response is attenuated, and the elderly increase their cardiac outputs by increasing stroke volume, rather than heart rate. To try to minimise all these effects, aim to ensure adequate, but not over-, hydration prior to induction, and try to avoid rapid swings in blood pressure during induction and subsequent maintenance of anaesthesia. Hence, intravenous induction of anaesthesia using propofol should be slow, titrating the dose to effect, remembering that the arm–brain circulation time may be greatly increased.
➤ In addition to the effects of normal ageing, there may be other pathology such as ischaemic heart disease.

Respiratory system:
➤ ↓ pulmonary elasticity.
➤ ↓ chest wall and lung compliance.
➤ ↓ TLC, FEV1, FVC, IRV.
➤ ↑ RV.
➤ FRC is not altered but closing capacity gradually encroaches on it, and will exceed it, when supine, from around 65 years old.
➤ Upper airway tone and the cough reflex decrease, causing an increased risk of obstruction and airway soiling.
➤ The elderly are more prone to infections and pulmonary emboli and the incidence of diseases such as COPD increases with age.

➤ In elective surgery it may be sensible to refer the patient to the physicians for pre-optimisation of any chest pathology.

Renal:

➤ The kidney's ability to both preserve and excrete water and electrolytes decreases.
➤ A reduction in muscle bulk is reflected in a decreased baseline creatinine.
➤ Careful attention to fluid balance, both peri and post-operatively, is required.
➤ It is sensible to avoid NSAIDs in those with pre-existing renal failure, and to limit their use to 3 days in those with normal renal function.
➤ Be aware that a modest rise in creatinine level may reflect a significant decline in renal function.

Central nervous system:

➤ The acuity of the special senses (sight, hearing) decreases with age. This can lead to difficulties in communicating, and can increase confusion in the elderly.
➤ Confusion and dementia increase with age and can be exacerbated by anaesthesia.
➤ Cerebrovascular disease is common.
➤ Avoid intraoperative hypotension which may result in cerebrovascular accident and attempt to avoid any centrally acting drugs that increase confusion where possible, e.g. atropine. It is sensible to try to recover confused patients in a quiet, calm, well-lit environment.

Musculoskeletal:

➤ Skin may be fragile. Extra care should be taken when moving the patient and attention to pressure areas to avoid the development of pressure sores.
➤ Arthritis is very common, and so care should be taken when positioning the anaesthetised patient so as not to cause pain in any affected joints. Pay special attention to neck mobility, especially in a patient with rheumatoid arthritis, looking specifically for the risk of atlanto-axial subluxation and a difficult airway.
➤ Balance, strength and postural reflexes worsen with age and so early mobilisation and physiotherapy is important to try to prevent significant loss of function in the post-operative period.

Pharmacology:

Pharmakokinetics can be altered due to:

➤ ↑ body fat and ↓ body water content.
➤ ↓ renal and liver blood flow.
➤ ↓ protein affects levels of free drug available.
➤ MAC ↓ with age.
➤ ↑ sensitivity to central depressants.
➤ Polypharmacy.
➤ Be aware of the need to be cautious with dosing drugs with narrow therapeutic indices, e.g. gentamicin. It may be necessary to decrease the dose, or increase the time between consecutive doses.

CHAPTER 38

Adrenal gland

Describe the anatomical organisation of the adrenal gland

The adrenal or suprarenal glands lie on top of the upper poles of the kidneys and play a key role in the synthesis of corticosteroids and catecholamines.

The adrenal glands are at the level of the twelfth thoracic vertebra. Anatomically, the adrenal gland is divided into two distinct areas: an outer cortex and inner medulla.

Adrenal cortex:
➤ Site of synthesis of corticosteroid hormones (glucocorticoids and mineralocorticoids) and androgens.
➤ Under neuroendocrine control via the hypothalamic – pituitary – adrenal axis.
➤ Part of the renin – angiotensin – aldosterone pathway.
➤ Divided into three functional zones from outside to inside: zona glomerulosa, zona fasiculata and zona reticularis (an easy way to remember this is 'GFR').

Adrenal medulla:
➤ Composed of chromaffin cells.
➤ Main site of synthesis of adrenaline and noradrenaline.
➤ Hormone secretion occurs in response to stimulation by pre-ganglionic (cholinergic) nerve fibres from the splanchnic nerves.

What are the main hormones secreted from each of the three zones of the adrenal cortex?
➤ **zona glomerulosa:** mineralocorticoids (aldosterone)
➤ **zona fasiculata:** glucocorticoids (cortisol)
➤ **zona reticularis:** androgens (dehydroepiandrosterone).

Describe the cortisol negative feedback pathway

The hypothalamus secretes corticotrophin-releasing hormone (CRH), which stimulates release of adrenocorticotrophic hormone (ACTH) from the anterior pituitary. ACTH stimulates cortisol secretion from the zona fasiculata of the adrenal cortex. Cortisol exerts negative feedback on both CRH and ACTH release.

Describe the control of aldosterone secretion
➤ **Renin-angiotensin-aldosterone (RAA) system:** Reduced circulating volume is detected by the reduction in renal afferent arteriolar pressure causing renin secretion from the juxtaglomerular cells. Renin cleaves angitensionogen to produce angiotensin I which is then converted to angiotensin II in the pulmonary vasculature by angiotensin-converting enzyme (ACE). Angiotensin II promotes aldosterone secretion.
➤ **Fall in plasma sodium concentration:** Reduced serum sodium is detected by the macula densa and stimulates the secretion of aldosterone in order to increase sodium retention.

➤ **Rise in plasma ACTH:** Also exerts a direct effect in increasing aldosterone secretion from the zona glomerulosa.

What are major actions of cortisol?

Cortisol exerts its effects by binding to glucocorticoid receptors and promoting specific enzyme synthesis. Cortisol has effects on metabolism, immune function and vascular reactivity:

➤ **Metabolism:**
  • increased protein catabolism
  • increased hepatic glycogenesis and gluconeogenesis
  • increased plasma glucose.
➤ **Vascular:**
  • cortisol is essential in maintaining vascular reactivity to noradrenaline.
➤ **Immune:**
  • suppresses the immune system and impairs wound healing.

What are the main actions of aldosterone?

Aldosterone increases the reabsorption of sodium from the distal convoluted tubules of the kidney, resulting in sodium retention and plasma expansion. It also increases urinary potassium excretion.

Describe how catecholamines are synthesised

Catecholamines are synthesised in the chromaffin cells of the adrenal medulla:

L-TYROSINE
↓ Tyrosine hydoxylase
L-DOPA
↓ Dopa decarboxylase
DOPAMINE
↓ Dopamine hydroxylase
NORADRENALINE
↓ Phenylethanolamine N-methyltransferase
ADRENALINE

CHAPTER 39

Pain pathways

Define and classify pain

Pain is 'an unpleasant sensory and emotional experience associated with actual or potential tissue damage' (IASP: International Association for the Study of Pain).

Pain can be classified according to its chronicity:

TABLE 1.48 Characteristics of acute versus chronic pain

Acute	Chronic
Recent onset, limited duration	Persists beyond time of healing or injury
Identifiable cause related to injury/disease	No clearly definable cause

It may also be classified according to its nature:
- **Nociceptive:** noxious stimulation of nociceptors. This may further be subdivided into:
  - superficial somatic pain (skin) – well-localised, sharp pain
  - deep somatic pain (ligaments, tendons, muscles) – dull, aching, poorly localised pain
  - visceral pain (organs, viscera) – cramping pain, varying localisation, associated with referred pain and autonomic stimulation.
- **Neuropathic:** due to dysfunction of the nervous system.

Give a detailed description of the pain pathways that become activated if you prick your finger with a pin

This is a mammoth question to answer! Consider starting your answer by drawing a simple diagram while explaining a brief overview of the main sites involved, and then going into greater detail later.
- Nociceptors respond to noxious stimuli, which may be thermal, mechanical or chemical.
- Tissue damage releases mediators, which initiate and sensitise receptor stimulation.
- An action potential is generated and propagated along the primary afferent nerve fibres (C and Aδ) to the dorsal horn of the spinal cord.
- Synaptic transmission with secondary interneurones occurs in Rexed's laminae.
- Secondary interneurones decussate and travel in the anterolateral spinothalamic tracts through the brainstem to the thalamus.
- From here, tertiary afferents project to the somatosensory cortex.
- Some spinal ascending fibres transmit impulses to the reticular activating system, and to higher centres involved with affect, emotion and memory.
- Descending fibres from cortex, thalamus and brainstem exert an inhibitory influence on pain transmission in the dorsal horn.
- An immediate polysynaptic withdrawal reflex occurs at the level of the spinal cord as some interneurones connect to motor neurones at many levels. This is a protective reflex.

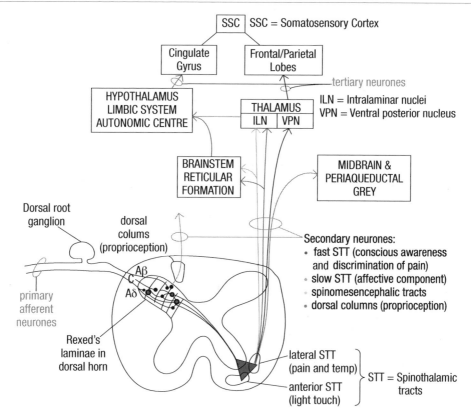

FIGURE 1.49 Schematic representation of pain pathways

What are nociceptors and how are they classified?

Pain receptors are unmyelinated nerve endings which are abundant in skin and musculoskel-etal tissue, and which respond to thermal, mechanical and chemical stimuli.

They are classified according to their sensitivity to the type of stimulus:

➤ **unimodal** (thermo-mechanoreceptors) respond to pinprick and sudden heat

➤ **polymodal** respond to pressure, heat, cold, chemicals and tissue damage.

How do noxious stimuli activate pain transmission?

➤ Chemical stimuli may be exogenous (e.g. capsaicin) or endogenous.

➤ Tissue injury causes damage to cell membranes and release of endogenous chemicals which stimulate nociceptors (bradykinin, histamine, serotonin, acetylcholine, H^+ and K^+ ions).

➤ Some chemical mediators lower the threshold for receptor stimulation, i.e. they sensitise nociceptors (prostaglandins, leukotrienes, substance P, neurokinin A and calcitonin gene-related peptide).

➤ Stimulation results in an influx of sodium and calcium ions, which cause depolarisation of the cell membrane and initiation of an action potential (AP).

➤ The AP is propagated along the nerve fibre (via sodium and calcium channels) to the dorsal root ganglion and the dorsal horn. The more heavily myelinated the nerve fibre is, the faster the impulse transmits.

➤ At the presynaptic terminal, the influx of calcium causes release of neurotransmitter into the synaptic cleft.

Which types of nerve fibres are involved?
➤ Three main types of fibres relay sensory inputs from the periphery (*see* Table 1.50).
➤ The cell bodies of all three fibres lie in the dorsal root ganglia.
➤ The fibres terminate in the dorsal horn of the spinal cord, where they synapse with secondary afferent neurones in Rexed's laminae.

TABLE 1.50 Characteristics of different nerve fibres

Afferent fibres	Aβ	Aδ	C
Stimulus	Non-noxious (pressure/touch)	Non-noxious and noxious (pain and temperature)	Polymodal noxious (mechanical, heat, chemical)
Diameter (μm)	Large, 6–20	Small, 2–5	Small, 0.4–1.2
Myelin	thick	thin	non
Conduction velocity (ms⁻¹)	80–120	12–30	0.5–2
Type of pain	Touch, pressure (no pain)	Fast, sharp, well-localised	Diffuse, dull
Dorsal horn termination (Rexed's laminae)	III	I (superficial) & V (deep)	II & III (substantia gelatinosa)

What happens at the level of the dorsal horn?
➤ The dorsal horn is the area of synaptic transmission between primary and secondary afferent neurones in Rexed's laminae.
➤ Laminae II and III are called the substantia gelatinosa where extensive modulation of pain occurs. It is the site of the 'gate control' theory of pain.

Describe the classes of second order neurones

TABLE 1.51 Classes of second order neurones

Class	Nociceptive-specific (NS)	Wide dynamic range (WDR)	Low-threshold neurones
Location	superficial laminae	deeper laminae	laminae III and IV
Response to type of stimulus	specific noxious	non-specific	innocuous
Synapse with primary fibre	C & Aδ	Aδ	Some Aβ

Which neurotransmitters and receptors are involved?
➤ The main excitatory neurotransmitters released by the primary afferent terminals include glutamate, aspartate and substance P ('gluta*mate* and aspar*tate* exci*tate!*'). These trigger various receptors on interneurones and secondary afferent neurones, such as:
- N-methyl D-aspartate (NMDA)
- α-amino-3-hydroxy-5-methylisoxazole-4-propionic acid (AMPA)
- neurokinin-1 (NK1)
- adenosine (A1/A2).

➤ Inhibitory neurotransmitters released locally include:
  - enkephalins (μ opioid receptors)
  - gamma-aminobutyric acid (GABA receptors).

Describe the path of the ascending spinal tracts to higher centres

There are multiple ascending tracts. The most important ones are:
➤ **Spinothalamic tracts (STT):** Most secondary fibres decussate and ascend as the anterolateral STT
  - anterior STT: light touch
  - lateral STT: pain and temperature.

  Fast (discriminatory) and slow (affective) fibres travel together to the brainstem where they separate to end in different nuclei.

  Fast fibres pass through the brainstem with no intermediary synapses before terminating in the **ventral posterior nucleus of the thalamus**. From here, tertiary neurones project to the **somatosensory cortex** (parietal and frontal lobes). They are responsible for conscious perception and memory of pain as well as its discrimination (location, intensity, quality).

  Slow (affective) fibres synapse in the brainstem's reticular formation and in intralaminar nuclei of the thalamus before projecting to the hypothalamus, limbic system and autonomic centres. Tertiary fibres project to the cingulate gyrus in the cortex. They are associated with the affective-arousal component of pain.
➤ **Spinoreticular tracts:** Slow fibres may also ascend in the spinoreticular tract, terminating in the reticular formation and thalamus.
➤ **Spinomesencephalic tracts:** These terminate in the midbrain and periaqueductal grey (PAG).
➤ **Dorsal columns:** Pressure, vibration and proprioception carried by Aβ fibres from the periphery ascend in the dorsal columns ipsilaterally. They do not transmit pain sensation to higher centres.

Describe the descending inhibitory pathways

➤ The **periaqueductal grey** (PAG) in the midbrain is the main descending pathway. It receives projections from the thalamus, hypothalamus, amygdala and cortex, and delivers projections to the nucleus raphe magnus (NRM) in the medulla, whose fibres synapse in the substantia gelatinosa of the dorsal horn. Its transmitters include endorphins and enkephalins (MOP receptors) and serotonin (5-HT$_1$ and 5-HT$_3$ receptors).
➤ The **locus caeruleus** (LC) is another important brainstem nucleus projecting descending inhibitory pathways to the dorsal horn via noradrenaline (α-adrenergic receptors).

What do you understand by the 'gate control' theory of pain modulation?

(Melzack and Wall 1965)

This is one aspect of pain modulation, reducing the response to nociceptive stimuli.

It postulates that pain transmission from primary to secondary afferents is 'gated' by interneurones in the substantia gelatinosa.

Inhibition can be presynaptic on primary afferents or postsynaptic on secondary afferent neurones.
➤ **Opening:** The 'gate' is opened presynaptically by C fibres via substance P ('pushes' the gate open) and postsynaptically by Aδ fibres, which inhibit the action of

enkephalinergic interneurones (which are inhibitory) at the level of the substantia gelatinosa.

➤ **Closure:** It is closed by descending inhibitory fibres, peripheral Aβ fibres and indirectly by the action of Aδ fibres on descending pathways.

Aβ fibres inhibit C fibre input presynaptically via stimulation of GABA receptors (which are inhibitory). Aβ fibres are stimulated by touch/pressure and explain how 'rubbing it better' and how high-frequency, low-amplitude TENS may attenuate pain.

Descending serotonergic (PAG, NRM) and noradrenergic (LC) fibres activate enkephalin-secreting interneurones which inhibit postsynaptic transmission. This explains how antidepressants (which block the reuptake of serotonin and noradrenaline) and opioids exert their effect.

Aδ fibres ascend and stimulate the PAG to exert its inhibitory action as above. This explains how acupuncture and how low-frequency TENS may attenuate pain.

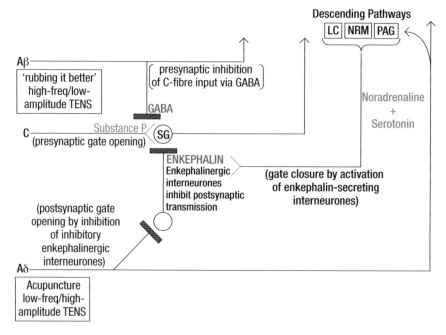

FIGURE 1.52 The 'gate control' theory of pain

Where are the sites of action of commonly used analgesic methods?

TABLE 1.53 Sites of action of analgesics

Analgesic	Site of action	Receptor	Neurotransmitter
Paracetamol	Central	+ 5-HT$_3$	+ serotonin
		+ cannabinoid	+ endogenous cannabinoids
	Peripheral	− COX	− prostaglandins
NSAIDs	nociceptor	− COX	− prostaglandins
Opiate	DH (presynaptic afferents)	+ MOP opioid	Reduced glutamate release from Aδ & C fibres (reduced nociceptive transmission)

Analgesic	Site of action	Receptor	Neurotransmitter
	PAG (postsynaptic secondary afferents)	– GABA receptor	– GABA (increased anti-nociceptive transmission)
Tramadol	DH	+ MOP opioid	Reduced glutamate release from Aδ & C fibres
	Descending pathways	+ 5-HT$_1$ & 5-HT$_3$ + α-adrenergic	+ presynaptic serotonin release and inhibition of reuptake of serotonin and noradrenaline
Antidepressants (TCAs)	Descending pathways: NRM LC	+ 5-HT$_1$ & 5-HT$_3$ + α-adrenergic	+ serotonin + noradrenaline (by inhibition of reuptake)
Anticonvulsants	Peripheral nerves	stabilise sodium channels	
Local anaesthetics	Peripheral nerve fibre	block sodium channels	
Ketamine	Dorsal horn secondary afferent	– NMDA	– glutamate
Clonidine	LC	+ α2-adrenergic agonist	+ noradrenaline
TENS	Aβ fibres 'closing the gate' in dorsal horn by presynaptic inhibition	+ GABA	+ GABA

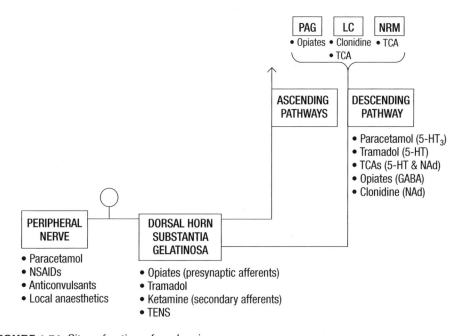

FIGURE 1.54 Sites of action of analgesics

CHAPTER 40

Thyroid gland

Describe the structure of the thyroid gland

The thyroid gland is a highly vascular structure made up of two lobes, joined together by the thyroid isthmus. The lobes are found on either side of the trachea, anterolaterally, below the larynx. The isthmus passes in front of the trachea overlying the second to fourth tracheal rings, in the adult.

At a cellular level, the gland is made up of thousands of follicles. Each of these is made up of a single layer of cells surrounding a cavity. These epithelial cells make thyroid hormones and secrete them into the cavity, where they are stored bound to thyroglobulin, which is a globular colloidal substance.

What are the thyroid hormones and how are they made?

There are three different thyroid hormones:

➤ thyroxine (T4)
➤ 3,5,3'-triiodothyronine (T3)
➤ 3,3,5'-triiodothyronine (reverse T3).

The majority of hormone synthesised is T4, but the active hormone is actually T3, which is five times more potent. T4 is converted to T3 peripherally to cause its biological effect. Reverse T3 is inactive.

T3/T4 are made as follows.

➤ The thyroid gland takes in iodine by active transport and concentrates it here.
➤ This iodine is oxidised to atomic iodine by peroxidase.
➤ The atomic iodine iodinates tyrosine residues found on the thyroglobulin molecule, to form mono– or di-iodotyrosine.
➤ These iodinated tyrosine residues then couple up to form either T3 or T4.
➤ The T3 and T4 hormones are stored as an integral part of the thyroglobulin molecule.

This process is driven by thyroid stimulating hormone (TSH) acting via cAMP. TSH also stimulates the release of the hormones by driving the endothelial cells to take in the colloidal thyroglobulin by pinocytosis. Once in the cell, proteolysis of the molecule causes release of T3 and T4. These diffuse into the ready blood supply and are transported out of the gland bound mainly to T4-binding globulin, but also to albumin and transthyretin.

What are the effects of the thyroid hormones?

T3, the major active hormone, exerts its effects by combining with a receptor in the cell nucleus and modulating protein synthesis at the level of the DNA. The actions of thyroid hormone can be divided into:

➤ **Metabolic**
  ↑ basal metabolic rate by increasing the rate of oxidative metabolism
  ↑ sensitivity to catecholamines
  ↑ breakdown of proteins, causing muscle wasting if unchecked
  ↑ turnover of calcium from bone.

➤ **Growth**
Needed for normal growth of tissues; by a direct effect and also a permissive effect on growth hormone.
➤ **Nervous system**
Needed for development of the nervous system normal myelination.
➤ **Others**
Needed for normal gonadal function and for lactation.

How are thyroid hormone levels controlled?
The hypothalamus produces thyroid-releasing hormone, which stimulates the release of TSH from the anterior pituitary. This in turn causes the release of T4/T3 from the thyroid gland. The T4/T3 released exerts a negative feedback effect on the hypothalamus and pituitary thereby reducing further release of stimulating hormones.

Ultimately, T4/T3 are broken down in the liver and most tissues. T4 has a half-life of around 1 week, while T3s is much shorter at around one day.

What are the symptoms and signs of hyperthyroidism?

TABLE 1.55 Symptoms of hyperthyroidism

System	Symptoms	Signs
CNS	Irritable, change in behavior, anxiety, eye changes, goitre	Tremor, restless, irritable, frank psychosis in severe cases, goitre, hyper-reflexia
		Eye signs: Exophthalmos (Graves'), lid lag, ophthalmoplegia
CVS	Palpitations, racing heart	Tachycardia, atrial fibrillation, hypertension, high output cardiac failure, warm and dilated peripheries
RS	Breathless	None specific
GI	Weight loss despite increased intake, vomiting, diarrhoea	Weight loss
GU	Loss of libido, gynaecomastia	Oligo/amenorrhea, gynaecomastia
Musculoskeletal	Weakness, tremor, fatigue	Proximal muscle wasting, tremor, palmar erythema, pretibial myxoedema

What are the symptoms and signs of hypothyroidism?

TABLE 1.56 Symptoms of hypothyroidism

System	Symptoms	Signs
CNS	Fatigue, slowness of thought	Flat affect, deafness, frank psychosis in severe cases, slow relaxing reflexes, ataxia
CVS	Ankle swelling	Bradycardia, ischaemic heart disease, peripheral oedema, low output cardiac failure, pericardial effusion (rare), hypertension, vasoconstricted and cold peripheries
RS	None	None
GI	Weight gain	Weight gain, constipation
GU	Menorrhagia	Infertility
Musculoskeletal	Thinning of hair, loss of eyebrows, dry skin	Proximal myopathy, muscular hypertrophy, myotonia

CHAPTER 41

Eye

Which cranial nerves supply the extraocular muscles?
Remember 'LR₆SO₄'.

➤ Lateral rectus muscle is supplied by the sixth cranial nerve (abducens nerve).
➤ Superior oblique muscle is supplied by the fourth cranial nerve (trochlear nerve).
➤ All of the other extraocular muscles (medial rectus, superior rectus, inferior rectus and inferior oblique) are supplied by the third cranial nerve (oculomotor nerve).

What determines intraocular pressure (IOP)?
Intraocular pressure is normally less than 15 mmHg. The effects of external pressure and the pressure exerted by intraocular contents determine intraocular pressure.

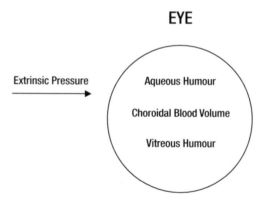

FIGURE 1.57 Schematic representation of the determinants of intraocular pressure

What are the causes of raised intraocular pressure?

➤ **Increased extrinsic pressure**, e.g. retrobulbar haematoma, orbital compression in the prone position.
➤ **Increased aqueous humour**, e.g. open-angle glaucoma (angle between iris and cornea remains patent but partially obstructed trabecular meshwork), closed-angle glaucoma (anterior bulging of the iris closing the drainage angle, trabecular meshwork remains patent).
➤ **Sulphur hexafluoride injection**, e.g. during retinal surgery SF6 may be injected into the vitreous. Nitrous oxide interacts with SF6 by increasing the volume of the gas and therefore may increase intraocular pressure.
➤ **Increased choroidal blood volume**, e.g. gravitational effects of head down position, hypoxia, hypercarbia, hypertension.

Describe the effects on intraocular pressure of the commonly used anaesthetic drugs
➤ **Induction agents** – all agents except for ketamine lower IOP.

➤ **Volatiles** – all lower IOP.
➤ **N$_2$O** – has no effect on IOP unless used in combination with surgical use of SF6 during vitreo-retinal surgery.
➤ **Neuromuscular blocking agents** – non-depolarising relaxants slightly lower IOP through reduction in extraocular muscle tension; suxamethonium causes a transient rise in IOP.

What is the oculocardiac reflex and how can it be prevented?

Oculocardiac reflex describes the bradycardia and or asystole observed as a result of traction on the extraocular muscles or extrinsic compression of the eye. The reflex pathway involves the trigeminal nerve and the vagus nerve. It is more pronounced in children. It may be obtunded by administration of anticholinergics such as atropine.

CHAPTER 42

Endothelium

What is the basic structure of endothelium?

Endothelium refers to the simple squamous epithelium that is found lining organs, blood vessels and body cavities. This single layer of cells lies on top of a basement membrane, and in small arteries, arterioles and glands it is also in close proximity to smooth muscle. Endothelial structure varies according to its site and function. The major types include:

➤ **Continuous endothelium** consists of a continuous basement membrane with endothelial cells anchored together via tight junctions. It has a low permeability and is found in the blood brain barrier and the lung.

➤ **Fenestrated endothelium** has pores (fenestrae) within the endothelium. It is very permeable and is found lining renal glomeruli.

➤ **Discontinuous endothelium** has large gaps between the endothelial cells and basement membrane. It is the most permeable of all types and is found in the liver and spleen.

What are the functions of endothelium?

Endothelium is a highly sophisticated and cellularly active tissue with essential roles in coagulation, inflammation and vasomotor tone. Its functions are varied and include the following:

➤ **Diffusion:** The endothelial lining at the alveolar-capillary interface plays an important role in the diffusion of gases (e.g. O_2 and CO_2) and lipid-soluble agents (e.g. anaesthetic drugs). The diffusion of such substances follows Fick's law.

➤ **Osmosis:** The endothelium lining the smaller blood vessels form a semi-permeable membrane, which allows the formation of interstitial fluid, based on Starling's forces.

➤ **Filtration:** The pores present within the endothelium of the Bowman's capsule permits the passage of fluid and electrolytes via bulk flow and thereby enables blood to be filtered.

➤ **Barrier:** In the blood brain barrier the tightly anchored endothelial cells form a relatively impermeable barrier that protects the central nervous system.

➤ **Vasomotor tone:** Endothelium releases several vasoactive substances that are crucial in regulating vascular smooth muscle tone. It produces nitric oxide (NO) from L-arginine in a reaction catalysed by nitric oxide synthetase. NO activates guanylate cyclase to produce cGMP, which causes vasodilatation. Endothelin-1 is another vasoactive substance produced by endothelial cells which causes vascular smooth muscle vasoconstriction.

➤ **Inflammation:** Vascular endothelium can synthesise several prostaglandins with prostacyclin (PGI_2) being the major derivative. PGI_2 promotes vasodilatation and inhibits platelet adhesion and therefore when vascular endothelium is damaged (e.g. atherosclerotic plaques) these vessels become prone to vasospasm and thrombosis.

➤ **Coagulation:** Endothelial damage exposes blood to tissue factor, which initiates the activation of the extrinsic clotting cascade.

➤ **Secretion:** Vascular endothelium, especially that lining the lungs, is rich in angiotensin-converting enzyme (ACE) which catalyses the conversion of angiotensin I to angiotensin II. This forms an important step in the renin-angiotensin-aldosterone system regulating blood pressure, sodium and water.

CHAPTER 43

Portal circulations

What is the definition of a portal circulation?

A portal circulation is one in which blood from the capillary bed of one organ structure drains into the capillary bed of another organ structure through a larger vessel, usually a vein or venule (hence they are also known as portal venous systems).

Can you name some portal circulations?

Examples of such circulations include the hepatic portal (*see* Chapter 21, 'Liver physiology'), placental, hypothalamo-hypophyseal and renal circulations.

Describe the hypothalamo-hypophyseal portal circulation

The hypothalamo-hypophyseal portal circulation allows hormones synthesised by the hypothalamic neurones to be transported rapidly and directly to the anterior pituitary to avoid dilution or destruction in the systemic circulation. These hormones diffuse into capillaries of the primary plexus located in the hypothalamus and are carried by hypophyseal portal veins (which run on the outside of the infundibulum) into the secondary capillary plexus of the anterior pituitary gland. These hypothalamic hormones either stimulate or inhibit the release of hormones from the anterior pituitary.

TABLE 1.58 Actions of hypothalamic hormones

Hypothalamic hormones	Effects on anterior pituitary hormones
Growth hormone-releasing hormone (GHRH)	Stimulates release of growth hormone (GH)
Somatostatin	Inhibits release of GH
Thyrotrophin-releasing hormone (TRH)	Stimulates release of thyroid-stimulating hormone
Gonadotrophin-releasing hormone (GnRH)	Stimulates release of follicle-stimulating hormone (FSH) and luteinising hormone (LH)
Corticotrophin-releasing hormone (CRH)	Stimulates release of adrenocorticotrophic hormone (ACTH) and melanocyte-stimulating hormone (MSH)
Prolactin-releasing hormone (PIH)	Stimulates release of prolactin

What are the functions of the anterior pituitary gland?

The anterior pituitary gland (also termed the adenohypophysis) secretes a host of hormones with wide-ranging effects. Once secreted, these hormones diffuse into the secondary capillary plexus and then into adenohypophyseal veins from where they get distributed to various target tissues.

TABLE 1.59 The effects of anterior pituitary hormones

Anterior pituitary hormone	Effect
GH	Stimulates liver to synthesise and release insulin-like growth factors (IGFs). These stimulate protein anabolism, lipolysis, tissue repair, cell growth and elevate plasma glucose levels.
TSH	Stimulates thyroid gland to release thyroxine (T4) and triiodothyronine (T3).
FSH	In females stimulates production of oocytes and secretion of ovarian oestrogen.
	In males stimulates sperm production.
LH	In females, stimulates ovulation, corpus luteum formation, secretion of ovarian oestrogen and secretion of corpus luteum progesterone.
	In males stimulates secretion of testicular testosterone.
ACTH	Stimulates release of glucocorticoids (mainly cortisol) from the adrenal cortex.
MSH	Stimulates darkening of skin.
Prolactin	Stimulates milk production.

Describe the renal portal circulation

The kidney is interesting because it contains two portal circulations. An afferent arteriole enters the Bowman's capsule and divides into multiple capillaries to form the glomerulus (this is the primary capillary bed). The efferent venule leaving the glomerulus enters two distinct secondary capillary beds: a capillary bed surrounding the cortical tubular system and a capillary bed surrounding the loop of Henle (the vasa recta). The function of these portal circulations is to maximise the reabsorption of water and electrolytes filtered at the glomerulus.

CHAPTER 44

Blood

Blood transfusion may be life saving, but it is not without risk. Many issues may be covered in an examination question including composition and storage of blood, risks and benefits of transfusion, effects of massive blood transfusion, infective and immunological effects of blood transfusion and blood conservation strategies.

Describe the composition and storage of blood

Whole blood is separated into red cells, plasma and platelets via centrifugation. Once separated plasma must be frozen as soon as possible to under −18°C, red cells must be stored at 1–6°C and platelets must be stored at room temperature (20–24°C) on shaking platforms (lifespan 3–5 days).

Leucodepletion is then performed in order to remove the white blood cells via filtration. Leucodeplete blood minimises the chances of alloimmunisation, reduces the incidence of febrile transfusion reactions and reduces the chances of cytomegalo virus (CMV) transmission.

Severely immunosuppressed patients require irradiated blood in order to prevent donor T-lymphocytes dividing in the recipient, which can result in transfusion and associated graft versus host disease. Stem cell transplant immunosuppressed patients will also require CMV negative blood.

The following changes occur in stored blood:
➤ fall in 2,3 DPG levels
➤ left shift of the oxyhaemoglobin dissociation curve
➤ fall in pH (approximately 7.0)
➤ rise in potassium concentration.

Storage solutions include:
➤ **Acid-citrate-dextrose:** Citrate acts as an anticoagulant by binding calcium while dextrose is an energy source for glycolysis. Red cell survival 21 days.
➤ **Citrate-phosphate-dextrose:** Increases red cell survival to 28 days.
➤ **Citrate-phosphate-dextrose-adenine:** The addition of adenine increases red cell ATP thereby increasing red cell survival to 35 days.
➤ **Saline (140 mmol/L)-adenine (1.5 mmol/L)-glucose (50 mmol/L)-mannitol (30 mmol/L):** Allows a greater volume of plasma to be removed from blood in order to use plasma for coagulation factors.

Discuss the risks and benefits of transfusion

The principal benefit of red cell transfusion is the improvement in oxygen-carrying capacity by increasing haemoglobin levels.

However, there are multiple risks and complications:
➤ **haemolytic transfusion reaction**, e.g. life-threatening ABO incompatibility versus delayed haemolysis to minor red cell antigens
➤ **febrile reactions**

- ➤ **infection transmission:** HIV (1 in 4 000 000), hepatitis A, hepatitis B, hepatitis c, malaria, variant CJD, CMV, syphilis, HTLV
- ➤ **metabolic:** hyperkalaemia and hypocalcaemia
- ➤ **hypothermia:** transfusion of cold stored blood
- ➤ **circulatory overload:** cardiac failure
- ➤ **immune:** graft versus host disease and possible increase in colorectal tumour recurrence rates
- ➤ **transfusion-related acute lung injury (TRALI):** incidence has fallen since the introduction of leucocyte deplete blood
- ➤ **iron overload** in chronic transfusion
- ➤ **septic shock** from bacterial contamination of donor blood.

What constitutes a massive transfusion?
There are many different definitions of what constitutes a massive transfusion but they all define a volume of transfusion and a time period, e.g. 10 units of blood within 6 hours or replacement of entire circulating volume with transfused blood within 24 hours.

The aim of treatment is the rapid and effective restoration of an adequate blood volume to maintain blood composition within safe limits with regards to haemostasis, oxygen-carrying capacity, oncotic pressure and biochemistry.

What are the problems encountered during massive transfusion?
Massive blood transfusion encompasses all of the risks of individual blood unit transfusion listed above but also has other specific problems:
- ➤ **Thrombocytopenia:** Dilutional thrombocytopenia is inevitable following massive transfusion as platelet function declines to zero after only a few days of storage. It has been shown that at least 1.5 times blood volume must be replaced for this to become a clinical problem. However, thrombocytopenia can occur following smaller transfusions if disseminated intravascular coagulation (DIC) occurs or there is pre-existing thrombocytopenia.
- ➤ **Coagulation factor depletion:** Stored blood contains all coagulation factors except V and VIII. Production of these factors is increased by the stress response to trauma. Therefore only mild changes in coagulation are due to the transfusion per se, and supervening DIC is more likely to be responsible for disordered haemostasis. DIC is a consequence of delayed or inadequate resuscitation, and the usual explanation for abnormal coagulation indices out of proportion to the volume of blood transfused.
- ➤ **Oxygen affinity changes:** Massive transfusion of stored blood with high oxygen affinity adversely affects oxygen delivery to the tissues. However, 2,3 DPG levels rise rapidly following transfusion and normal oxygen affinity is usually restored in a few hours.
- ➤ **Hypocalcaemia:** Each unit of blood contains approximately 3 g citrate, which binds ionised calcium. The healthy adult liver will metabolise 3 g citrate every 5 minutes. Transfusion at rates higher than one unit every 5 minutes or impaired liver function may thus lead to citrate toxicity and hypocalcaemia. Hypocalcaemia does not have a clinically apparent effect on coagulation, but patients may exhibit transient tetany and hypotension. Calcium should only be given if there is biochemical, clinical or electrocardiographic evidence of hypocalcaemia.
- ➤ **Hyperkalaemia:** The plasma potassium concentration of stored blood increases during storage and may be over 30 mmol/L. Hyperkalaemia is generally not a problem unless very large amounts of blood are given quickly. On the contrary, hypokalaemia is more

common as red cells begin active metabolism and intracellular uptake of potassium restarts.

➤ **Acid–base disturbances:** Lactic acid levels in the blood pack give stored blood an acid load of up to 30–40 mmol/L. This, along with citric acid, is usually metabolised rapidly. Indeed, citrate is metabolised to bicarbonate, and a profound metabolic alkalosis may ensue. The acid–base status of the recipient is usually of more importance, final acid–base status being dependent on tissue perfusion, rate of administration and citrate metabolism.

➤ **Hypothermia:** Leads to reduction in citrate and lactate metabolism (leading to hypocalcaemia and metabolic acidosis), increase in affinity of haemoglobin for oxygen, impairment of red cell deformability, platelet dysfunction and an increased tendency to cardiac dysrhythmias.

➤ **Acute respiratory distress syndrome (ARDS):** The aetiology of ARDS is as yet not fully understood, but various risk factors have been identified. Both under– and over-transfusion are associated with an increased risk of ARDS, as is albumin < 30 g/L. Microaggregate filters should be used during massive transfusion except when giving fresh whole blood or platelets.

During massive blood transfusion, specific component therapy is required, namely FFP 12 mL/kg to provide coagulation factors, platelets (keep count > 50 000), cryoprecipitate for fibrinogen replacement (if fibrinogen < 1.0 g/L). Recent research from the military suggests empiric administration of FFP (in a ratio of 1:1 with blood, platelets and cryoprecipitate) may be prudent in the setting of massive bleeding and transfusion, rather than waiting for laboratory blood counts and coagulation test results.

What blood conservation strategies are available?
Remembering that blood transfusion can be associated with morbidity and mortality, there exist a number of strategies with the aim of reducing the need for transfusion.

➤ **Restrictive red cell transfusion trigger** – Accepting a lower haemoglobin level which is safe for the individual patient, e.g. 10 g/dL for a patient with ischaemic heart disease and possibly as low as 7 g/dL for a fit 20 year old.

➤ **Pre-donation** – Patients for planned surgery with significant expected blood loss may be candidates for pre-donation of blood followed by intraoperative transfusion of their own blood.

➤ **Hypotensive anaesthesia** – Used in certain types of surgery such as middle ear surgery or neurosurgery to reduce blood loss.

➤ **Anti-fibrinolytic agents** – Tranexamic acid and aprotinin inhibit clot breakdown.

➤ **Intraoperative blood salvage via cell savers** – Used in certain types of surgery.

➤ **Recombinant factor VII** – Used in haemophilia and in massive bleeding, provided platelet count is adequate (not effective in the setting of thrombocytopenia).

➤ **Artificial oxygen carriers** – Perflurocarbons and modified haemoglobins are the two main products. Oxygen transport characteristics of perfluorocarbon emulsions are fundamentally different from those of blood. Blood exhibits a sigmoidal oxygen dissociation curve. In contrast, perfluorocarbon emulsions are characterised by a linear relationship between oxygen partial pressure and oxygen content. Elevated arterial oxygen partial pressures are thus beneficial to maximise the oxygen transport capacity of perfluorocarbon emulsions. No artificial oxygen carriers are used extensively within the UK at present.

CHAPTER 45

Muscle electrophysiology

What is the resting membrane potential of a skeletal muscle cell?
Resting membrane potential for skeletal muscle is –90 mV, nervous tissue is –70 mV and cardiac muscle is –90 mV.

Describe the anatomical structure of a skeletal muscle
A skeletal muscle is covered by a connective tissue called the epimysium. Within the muscle lie thousands of muscle fibres, which are arranged in bundles or fascicles, surrounded by perimysium. These muscle fibres are cylindrical shaped, multi-nucleated cells, 10–100 μm in diameter and run along the entire length of the muscle. They are surrounded by endomysium.

Microscopically, muscle fibres have a striated appearance due to the presence of numerous myofibrils. The myofibrils are formed by thick (myosin) and thin (actin) contractile filaments in association with the regulatory proteins tropomyosin and troponin. These contractile filaments are arranged within sarcomeres, which form the basic contractile unit of a skeletal muscle.

What are the major components of the neuromuscular junction?
Neuromuscular transmission occurs across the neuromuscular junction, which is comprised of the α-motor neurone, synaptic cleft and motor end plate of the muscle fibre.

The end terminals of the motor neurone are unmyelinated, with specialised sites for the storage and release of acetylcholine (ACh). The motor end plate of the muscle fibre is deeply folded, with high concentrations of nicotinic acetylcholine receptors (nAChR) located at the crests of these folds. Separating these two components is the synaptic cleft, a 20 μm gap containing acetylcholinesterase.

How is acetylcholine synthesised and stored within the nerve terminal?
ACh is synthesised within the axoplasm from choline (obtained from the diet and liver synthesis) and acetyl coenzyme A (a metabolic by-product) in a reaction catalysed by choline-O-acetyltransferase. Once formed, approximately 80% is stored in vesicles available for release. Some of these vesicles (about 1%) lie at special release sites known as 'active zones' and are available for immediate release, while the others form the 'reserve pool', and are ready for transportation to the release site when needed. A remaining 20% forms a 'stationary store' dissolved in the cytoplasm.

How does neuromuscular transmission occur?
When a motor nerve is depolarised, voltage-gated Ca^{2+} channels open in the presynaptic membrane, allowing Ca^{2+} to enter the nerve terminal. This Ca^{2+} enables the vesicles to fuse and release their contents, it is believed, by exocytosis.

Approximately 100–200 vesicles simultaneously release their ACh, producing an end plate potential. When ACh binds to nAChR (pentameric, ligand-gated ion-channels consisting of 2α, 1β, 1ε and 1γ subunits) the receptor undergoes a conformational change and the central ion channel opens sufficiently to allow the passage of cations, predominantly Na^+ and K^+. This causes a localised depolarisation of the muscle fibre membrane, which leads to excitation-contraction coupling. The action of ACh is rapidly terminated by the presence of acetylcholinesterase within the synaptic cleft.

When do extra-junctional nAChR appear?

Extra-junctional nAChR rapidly sprout after denervation and burns injuries. These receptors are structurally different as the normal ε subunit is replaced by the fetal γ subunit. They are extremely sensitive to depolarising neuromuscular blocking agents and the use of these agents can result in profound hyperkalaemia. This is why suxamethonium is typically contraindicated in such patients from 24 hours to 2 years after injury. In contrast, extra-junctional receptors are relatively resistant to non-depolarising neuromuscular blocking agents and therefore these drugs must be administered at higher doses.

Describe the positive feedback mechanism designed to increase ACh release

There are pre-junctional nAChR located on the nerve terminals, which form a positive feedback mechanism designed to increase the release of ACh during periods of high activity (e.g. tetanic stimulation). These receptors are blocked by non-depolarising neuromuscular blocking drugs and this explains why fade on train-of-four stimulation is observed with these agents.

What is a motor unit?

A motor unit refers to a single motor neurone and all the muscle fibres it innervates. In muscles involved in fine, precise movement (e.g. eyes and fingers) the motor units are small and one motor neurone innervates only a few muscle fibres. This is in sharp contrast to muscles involved in gross, powerful movement where the motor unit consists of a single neurone innervating hundreds of fibres (e.g. quadriceps muscle).

What is excitation-contraction coupling?

This refers to the process by which the electrical activity of muscle depolarisation results in mechanical changes leading to contraction.

As the action potential travels down the T-tubules, which lie in very close proximity to the sarcoplasmic reticulum, it triggers calcium release channels (i.e. the ryanodine receptors) on the sarcoplasmic reticulum to open resulting in an influx of intracellular Ca^{2+}. This Ca^{2+} binds onto troponin, bringing about a conformational change in the troponin-tropomyosin complex, which results in the exposure of the myosin binding sites on the actin filaments. The myosin heads bind to actin, and perform a ratchet-type movement towards the centre of the sarcomeres, dubbed 'the power stroke'. ATP then binds onto the myosin head, allowing it to detach from the actin. The hydrolysis of this ATP enables the myosin head to re-orientate itself ready for the next power stroke. The muscle relaxes when intracellular Ca^{2+} levels decrease.

Rigor mortis occurs due to the lack of ATP, which prevents the detachment of the myosin heads from actin and hence the filaments are held in sustained contraction.

In malignant hyperpyrexia there is a defect in the ryanodine receptor which leads to the uncontrolled release of Ca^{2+} from within the sarcoplasmic reticulum and hence the sustained muscle contraction and rigidity seen in this condition.

CHAPTER 46

Reflexes

What are reflexes?

Reflexes are neuronal pathways that produce rapid, automatic and predictable responses to a stimulus. The basic components of the reflex arc include a receptor, afferent sensory neurone, synapse, efferent motor neurone and effector organ.

When we talk about reflexes we typically think of somatic reflexes, e.g. knee jerk stretch reflex, which are important in the functioning of the skeletal muscle system. However, equally important are the visceral reflexes, e.g. pupillary light reflex, which form the basis of the functioning of the autonomic nervous system.

What is the Bell–Magendie law?

This law states that the anterior spinal nerve roots contain only motor fibres and the posterior nerve roots contain only sensory fibres.

Describe the physiology of the stretch reflex

The stretch reflex (e.g. knee jerk stretch reflex) is a monosynaptic reflex that results in the contraction of a muscle in response to its being stretched.

Muscle spindle receptors within the muscle are stimulated when the muscle fibres are stretched, resulting in the generation of a potential. Provided this is of sufficient magnitude, an action potential is generated and propagates down afferent sensory neurones (Ia and II) to enter the grey matter of the spinal cord. They synapse within the ventral horn with efferent motor neurones (Aα), which project back to the extrafusal muscle fibres of the stretched muscle and cause it to contract. The sensory neurones also synapse with inhibitory inter-neurones, which innervate the antagonistic muscle group. Hence when the stretched muscle contracts during the reflex, its antagonistic muscles relax. This is known as reciprocal innervation. Stretch reflexes help maintain muscle tone, aid posture and prevent injury by opposing overstretching of muscles.

What is the inverse stretch reflex?

This refers to the relaxation of a muscle in response to a strong stretch. The harder a muscle is stretched, the more forcefully it will contract. However, there comes a point when muscle tension becomes so great that the Golgi tendon organs detect this and inhibit the activity of the efferent Aα motor neurones via an inhibitory feedback mechanism. This system is designed to prevent muscle damage.

Describe the physiology of the withdrawal (flexor) reflex

This is an important reflex governing the response to a painful stimulus and is an example of a polysynaptic reflex. Nociceptors are stimulated and impulses are propagated along sensory Aδ and C fibres into the grey matter of the spinal cord. Here they synapse with inter-neurones that extend to several spinal cord segments. These inter-neurones activate various Aα motor neurones, which culminate in the contraction of the flexor muscles of the effected limb. However, in order to maintain balance during a sudden flexor withdrawal of a lower limb, the pain stimulus also activates a cross-extensor reflex, which results in the automatic extension of the contralateral limb.

How are nerve fibres classified?

Classification of nerve fibres has become confusing with the use of both alphabetical and numerical classification systems. Originally, mammalian nerves were classified alphabetically into A, B or C fibre types. The A fibre type was then further subdivided into α, β, γ and δ groups. However, as science evolved it became apparent that the alphabetical classification system was inadequate because not all nerve fibre types within the originally assigned group were the same. Therefore, a numerical system was introduced to classify sensory neurones.

TABLE 1.60 Classification of nerve fibres

Fibre type	Axon diameter (μm)	Velocity (m/s)	Function
Aα	10–20	60–120	Motor
Aβ	5–10	40–70	Touch
			Pressure
Aγ	3–6	15–30	Motor to muscle spindles
Aδ	2–5	10–30	Pain
			Temperature
B	1–3	3–15	Autonomic (pre-ganglionic)
C	0.5–1	0.5–2	Pain
			Temperature
Ia (Aα type)	12–20	72–120	Sensory from muscle spindle (annulospiral)
Ib (Aα type)	12–20	72–120	Sensory from Golgi tendon
II (Aβ type)	4–12	24–72	Sensory from muscle spindle (flower-spray)
III (Aδ type)	1–4	6–24	Pain Cold
IV (C type)	0.5–1	0.5–2	Pain Temperature

2
Physics

CHAPTER 47

Definitions

A lot of physics SOE will start with a definition, which will then lead on to more detailed questioning on the surrounding concepts. This list is by no means exhaustive and should you encounter other definitions it is worthwhile making note of them.

Absolute humidity: Mass of water vapour present in a given volume of air (does not change with temperature). Measured in kgm^{-3}.

Absolute zero: Temperature at which all molecular motion stops ($0\,K$ or $-273.16°C$).

Ampere (A): SI unit of current. The current which produces a force of $2 \times 10^{-7}\,Nm^{-1}$ between 2 parallel wires, of infinite length, $1\,m$ apart in a vacuum. $1\,A = 1$ coulomb/s.

Boiling point: Temperature at which the vapour pressure of a liquid equals the surrounding ambient pressure.

Calorie: Amount of energy required to increase the temperature of $1\,g$ of water by $1°C$ (1 calorie $= 4.16\,J$).

Candela (cd): The SI unit of luminous intensity. 1 cd is the luminous intensity, in a given direction, of a source that emits monochromatic radiation of frequency 540×10^{12} hertz and that has a radiant intensity in that direction of $1/683$ watt per steradian.

Coulomb (C): Unit of charge. $1\,C$ is the amount of charge passing a given point per second, when $1\,A$ of current is flowing. $1\,C$ is the magnitude of charge possessed by 6.24×10^{18} electrons.

Critical temperature: Temperature above which a gas cannot be liquefied by pressure alone.

Freezing point: Temperature at which the liquid and solid phases of a substance of specified composition are in equilibrium at a given pressure.

Force: That which changes a body's state of rest or motion.

Gas: Gaseous substance above its critical temperature.

Heat capacity: Amount of energy required to raise the temperature of the whole body by $1°C$ (specific heat capacity × mass of body).

Hertz (Hz): SI unit of frequency. $1\,Hz$ is 1 cycle per second.

Joule (J): SI unit of energy. $1\,J$ is the work done (or energy expended) when the application of a $1\,N$ force moves $1\,m$ in the direction of the force ($1\,J = 1\,N \times 1\,m$).

Kelvin (K): SI unit of temperature. $1\,K$ is equal to $1/273.16$ of the thermodynamic scale temperature of the triple point of water.

Kilogram (kg): SI unit of mass. The standard kilogram is the mass of a cylindrical piece of platinum-iridium alloy kept in Sèvres, France.

Kinetic energy: Energy of motion of a body, equal to the work it would do if it were brought to rest.

Latent heat: Heat energy required when a substance changes phase at a given temperature.

Latent heat of fusion: Amount of heat required to convert a unit mass of a solid at its melting point into a liquid without an increase in temperature.

Latent heat of vaporisation: Amount of heat required to convert a unit mass of a liquid at its boiling point into vapour without an increase in temperature.

Mass: Amount of matter contained in a body. It does not alter under conditions of differing gravity (unlike weight).

Metre (m): SI unit of length. Originally the length of a platinum-iridium bar kept near Paris, but doubts existed as to the bar's length changing over time. Now defined according to the speed of light in a vacuum such that the speed of light is exactly 299,792,458 ms^{-1}.

Mole: SI unit of amount of substance. Quantity containing the same number of particles as there are atoms in 12 g of carbon–12. This number of particles (6.022×10^{23}) is known as Avogadro's number.

Momentum: Mass × velocity.

Newton (N): SI unit of force. 1 N is the force required to accelerate a mass of 1 kg by 1 ms^{-2}.

Ohm (Ω): Unit of electrical resistance. Resistance between two points on a conductor when a constant potential difference of 1 V between them produces a current of 1 A.

Pascal (Pa): 1 Pa is the force of 1 N acting over 1 m^2.

pH: Negative logarithm to the base 10 of hydrogen ion concentration in a solution. $pH = -\log_{10}[H^+]$.

Potential energy: Energy of a body or system as a result of its position in an electric, magnetic or gravitational field. It is the potential to do work.

Power: Rate of energy expenditure.

Pressure: Force per unit area. SI unit is the Pascal.

Relative humidity: Ratio of the mass of water in a given volume of air in relation to the mass of water vapour it could hold if fully saturated at a given temperature. Given as a percentage, it is equal to vapour pressure/saturated vapour pressure.

Resistance: Property of a conductor to oppose the flow of current through it.

Saturated vapour pressure (SVP): Pressure exerted by a vapour when in contact with and in equilibrium with its liquid phase within a closed system.

Second (s): SI unit of time. Defined according to the frequency of radiation emitted by caesium–133 in its ground state.

Specific heat capacity (SHC): Amount of energy required to raise the temperature of 1 kg of a substance by 1°C (SHC of water = 4.16 J and SHC of human body = 3.5 kJ).

Specific latent heat of vaporisation (SLHV): Energy required to change 1 kg of liquid into vapour (SLHV of water at 37.5°C is 2420 kJ/kg and SLHV of water at 100°C is 2260 kJ/kg).

Triple point of water: Conditions in which water exists in equilibrium in all three phases (occurs at a pressure of 0.006 atm and 0.01°C).

Vapour: Gaseous substance below its critical temperature.

Volt (V): Unit of electrical potential. 1 V is the potential difference between two points when 1 J of work is done to move 1 C of charge across them. 1 V will 'push' a current of 1 A through a resistance of 1 Ω.

Watt (W): SI unit of power. $1 W = 1 Js^{-1}$

Weight: Gravitational force acting on an object. It is the product of mass × gravitational acceleration ($9.81 ms^{-2}$). A mass of 1 kg will therefore have 9.81 N acting on it.

CHAPTER 48

Standard international units

The creation of the decimal metric system began during the eighteenth-century French revolution when two platinum standards, representing the metre and kilogram, were placed in the Archives de la Republique in Paris. Eminent scientists like Gauss and Weber then went on to promote the universal application of a standard system of measurement in the early nineteenth-century. By the 1960s, the International System of Units (abbreviated to SI units from the French *Le Système International d'Unités*) was developed which incorporated six base units (the mole was added later) along with rules for the use of derived units and prefixes. The advantage of this unified system is that equations and calculations will produce answers in the appropriate SI unit, but unfortunately not everyone uses them.

It is a popular opening question in the physics SOE and candidates should understand the relationship between derived and base units and be comfortable in manipulating them from one to the other.

What are the fundamental (base) units?
There are seven base units, which are considered to be dimensionally independent.

TABLE 2.1 Base units

Base unit	Name	Symbol
Length	metre	m
Mass	kilogram	kg
Time	second	s
Current	ampere	A
Temperature	kelvin	K
Amount of substance	mole	mol
Luminous intensity	candela	cd

What are the two supplementary units?
The plane angle (radian) and solid angle (steradian) were supplementary units but this category was abolished in 1995. These units are considered named derived units.

Can you list some of the derived units?
Derived units are formed by combination of various base units according to mathematical relationships, which link these quantities.

TABLE 2.2 Derived units

Derived units	Name	Symbol
Area	square metre	m^2
Volume	cubic metre	m^3
Density	kilogram per cubic metre	kg/m^3
Velocity	metre per second	m/s
Acceleration	metre per second squared	m/s^2

Can you list some named derived units?
These are derived units that have been given specific names.

TABLE 2.3 Named derived units

Named derived unit	Name (Symbol)	Expression in terms of other SI units	Expression in terms of base SI units
Force	newton (N)	–	$kg.m.s^{-2}$
Pressure	pascal (Pa)	N/m^2	$kg.m^{-1}.s^{-2}$
Energy	joule (K)	$N.m$	$kg.m^2.s^{-2}$
Power	watt (W)	J/s	$kg.m^2.s^{-3}$
Electric charge	coulomb (C)	–	$A.s$
Electric potential difference	volt (V)	W/A	$kg.m^2.s^{-3}.A^{-1}$
Capacitance	farad (F)	C/V	$kg^{-1}.m^{-2}.s^4.A^2$
Electrical resistance	ohm (Ω)	V/A	$kg.m^2.s^{-3}.A^{-2}$
Magnetic flux	weber (Wb)	$V.s$	$kg.m^2.s^{-2}.A^{-1}$
Magnetic flux density	tesla (T)	Wb/m^2	$kg.s^{-2}.A^{-1}$
Inductance	henry (H)	Wb/A	$kg.m^2.s^{-2}.A^{-2}$
Temperature	degree celsius (°C)	–	$K-273.15$

What are the common prefixes used for SI units?
Prefixes are decimal (base 10) multiples and submultiples of the quantity.

TABLE 2.4 Prefixes used for SI units

Prefix name (Symbol)	Multiple	Prefix name (Symbol)	Multiple
deca (da)	10^1	deci (d)	10^{-1}
hecto (h)	10^2	centi (c)	10^{-2}
kilo (k)	10^3	milli (m)	10^{-3}
mega (M)	10^6	micro (μ)	10^{-6}
giga (G)	10^9	nano (η)	10^{-9}
tera (T)	10^{12}	pico (p)	10^{-12}
peta (P)	10^{15}	femto (f)	10^{-15}
exa (E)	10^{18}	atto (a)	10^{-18}
zetta (Z)	10^{21}	zepto (z)	10^{-21}
yotta (Y)	10^{24}	yocto (y)	10^{-24}

CHAPTER 49

Principles of measurement

Describe the components of a standard measurement system

Measurement systems are used to detect an input, transduce the signal and display it in a form that can be used by an interpreter.

They are made up of the following:

➤ **Input** – parameter chosen to be measure, e.g. blood pressure (BP).
➤ **Transducer** – device that converts one form of energy into another, e.g. the strain gauge inside an invasive BP monitoring transducer. The pressure generated by the arterial pulse alters the shape of the diaphragm on which strain gauges are arranged as a Wheatstone bridge. The deformation alters the length of the wire in the gauges and so their resistance alters. The change in electrical signal is fed via the transmission path into the conditioning unit.
➤ **Transmission path** – apparatus that carries the electrical signal to the conditioning unit.
➤ **Conditioning unit** – apparatus in which the electrical signal is processed, analysed and then passed to the display unit.
➤ **Display unit** – monitor, gauge or dial on which the output is displayed.
➤ **Output** – final stage, and what is viewed on the screen, dial or gauge. The clinical context and the limitations of the equipment used must be taken into consideration when interpreting the output.

Measurement systems can either be **analogue** or **digital**.

➤ **Analogue** – output signal is continuous, e.g. the waveform display of an arterial pressure trace.
➤ **Digital** – output signal is discontinuous, e.g. the numerical display of BP next to the arterial waveform.

Which factors affect the output of a measurement system?

➤ **Accuracy** – this determines how closely the output reflects the true value being measured. Machines have their accuracy quoted in percentage by the manufacturers, e.g. a machine that displayed 110 units when the true value was 100 would have an accuracy of +/−10% across its working range.
➤ **Sensitivity** – this determines how small a change in input will result in a change in output. Less sensitive systems will be able to operate over a wider range.
➤ **Drift** – as the name suggests, this is a movement of the output away from the true input value. It is usually linear and unidirectional (though it does not have to be). It is usually caused by changing properties of the components of the equipment, e.g. ageing of thermistors.
➤ **Gain** – this refers to the degree of amplification of the measurement system (i.e. the output to input ratio).

What is hysteresis?

In a system with hysteresis, the output of the system alters depending on whether the input is rising or falling. In a system without hysteresis the output can be predicted from the input alone, but with hysteresis the operator needs to know the input history to estimate the output. An example of this is seen in the lung compliance curve, which exhibits hysteresis because of the elastic energy that is stored within it.

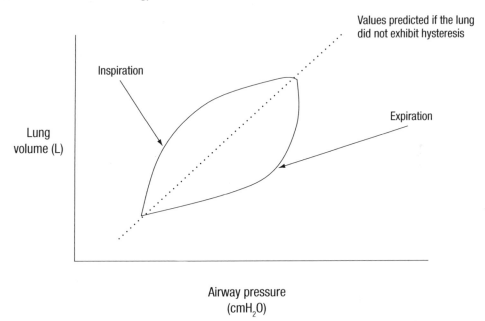

GRAPH 2.5 Lung volume-pressure (compliance) curve showing hysteresis

What is damping?

This is definitely an answer to practise aloud before you go into the exam. Although it is intuitively simple to understand, damping can be surprisingly hard to explain. We think it is easiest to draw the next graph (Graph 1.6) and use it to illustrate your answer.

In the perfect measurement system, any change in input would be instantly and accurately reflected in the output. However, this is not the case in clinical systems and it takes time for a change in input to be reflected by a change in output. The speed with which this happens can be measured and defined:

➤ The '**response time**' is the time taken for the output to reach 90% of its final reading.

➤ The '**rise time**' is the time taken for the output to rise from 10 to 90% of its final reading.

Though it is impossible to design the 'perfect' system described above, we do want a system, which responds as rapidly as possible to any change in input. This in itself can create problems, as a system which rises quickly will have the tendency to overshoot in its reading, while one which rises too slowly may never reach the new elevated input value, or may simply take too long to be a useful measure of a changing input.

➤ **Damping** describes the resistance of a system to oscillation, which results from a change in the input. Damping is the result of frictional forces working in that system.

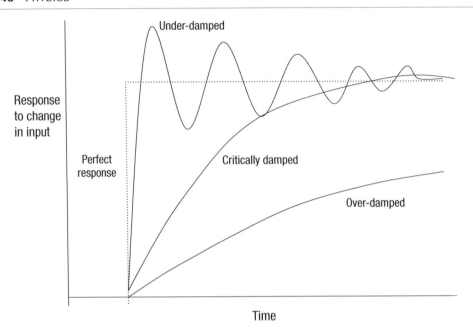

GRAPH 2.6 Damping

So, following a change in input there are four possible outcomes for the system:
➤ **Perfect response** – described above.
➤ **Under-damped** – the output changes quickly in response to the step up in input, but it overshoots and then oscillates around the true value, before coming to rest at it. This means that it will be some time before the true value is displayed and the peaks and troughs will over and under represent the true value. In a dynamic system, e.g. intra-arterial BP, the constantly changing input may result in wild fluctuations, rendering an under-damped system very inaccurate (although the MAP is still correct).
➤ **Over-damped** – the output here changes so slowly that it may never reach the true value. In a dynamic system, the response time may be simply too slow for the system to be useful.
➤ **Critically damped** – this is the best compromise for the system. The response and rise time of the system are longer than an under-damped response, but there is no significant overshoot and oscillations are minimal. 'D' is the damping factor and, by convention, in a critically damped system **D = 1**.

In reality in clinical measurement systems, critical damping is not ideal. We are prepared to accept a few oscillations and some overshoot for a faster response time. Hence, our systems are 'optimally damped' where 64% of the energy is removed from the system and **D = 0.64**. There is a 7% overshoot in this case.

What are the characteristics of the ideal invasive BP monitoring equipment?
➤ A short, stiff, wide cannula. This helps to keep its natural frequency high (*see* explanation below).
➤ No connections in the system, again to keep the natural frequency high.
➤ No air bubbles in the system as these are compressible and therefore decrease energy transmission up the column of fluid resulting in a damped trace.

What is calibration?

Calibration is a process in which the output of a measuring device is compared to a standard of known units of measure, to determine the accuracy of the measuring device. For example, a blood gas machine may be primed with a solution of known pH and its output compared with the known value of the solution. If the measuring device is proved to be inaccurate it can be reset accordingly.

Calibration should not be done against just one standard; at least two must be used. The more standards that are used for comparison, the more accurate will be the resultant measuring device.

Calibration should be performed when:

➤ A predetermined period of time has elapsed.
➤ The machine has been used a predetermined number of times.
➤ The machine gives unexpected results.
➤ The machine is moved, undergoes vibration or damage.

What is 'signal noise'?

Signal noise describes unwanted external information that is fed unintentionally into a transducer, resulting in the output being altered. We see this on the ECG display when diathermy is being used. Often here, the noise is so 'loud' that it actually obscures the ECG display. The magnitude of noise is described by comparing the two amplitudes to give the 'Signal: Noise (S/N) ratio'.

How can we overcome noise?

➤ We can add 'filters' into measurement systems, so that signals above or below given frequencies are 'ignored' and not processed to produce an output.
  • High pass filters ignore signals below a given frequency.
  • Low pass filters ignore signals above a given frequency.
  • Notch filters ignore signals at a given frequency, e.g. 50 Hz – mains frequency.
➤ We can average out the signal in cases where the signal is repetitive (as in most biological systems) and the noise is intermittent. This is useful when the noise is very loud compared to the desired signal.

Resonance and natural frequency

Resonance is the tendency of a system to oscillate at maximum amplitude at certain frequencies. This resonant frequency is determined by the mass and stiffness of the system. The greater the mass, the slower the oscillations, and the stiffer the system, the faster the oscillations.

The components of a measurement system will oscillate at their own natural frequency. Imagine that we are able to give energy to the system at the perfect moment to allow us to increase the amplitude of these oscillations. As the oscillations got bigger, it would be impossible to stop them being transmitted to the output reading. In this way, the *method* of measuring the true value would interfere with the output value displayed. For the 'physics challenged' among us, an easier way to visualise this is to imagine yourself on a swing. If you push off, and swing your legs at a steady rate, your swinging, or oscillation, will remain fairly constant. If, however, a friend comes and pushes you when you are at your highest point, they give energy to your system and you will swing higher and higher – your oscillations will increase in amplitude. If you were attached to an output monitor, you would see the units displayed increase. The key to this concept is that your friend has to push you at just the right point in your swing; too soon or too late, and they will not help increase your amplitude, and may even decrease it.

For our clinical example, think of the invasive BP transducer. If its natural frequency was near that of the input being measured (i.e. the swings up and down of the arterial pulse) it is easy to see how its own natural oscillations could be augmented by those of the pulse, which could act like the friend pushing the swing. The natural frequency of the arterial pulse is around 20 Hz (because it is comprised of lots of sine waves 'stacked' on top of each other, each with a frequency of approximately 2 Hz). For this reason, the manufacturers try to make the natural frequency of the transducer kit out of this range, and in fact most kits have a natural frequency of around 45 000 Hz.

This would work well, were it not for the way we then choose to use the carefully designed apparatus. We do not have the transducer in close proximity to the artery; instead we attach a long column of saline to the end of the transducer and attach this to the arterial cannula. This is for convenience, but it dramatically reduces the natural frequency of the measuring system. The long, heavy saline column reduces the natural frequency from 45 000 Hz to around 15 Hz and this brings the frequency of the measuring system very close to that of the input. Hence, it is now easy to see how the oscillations in BP can augment the oscillations of the measuring system and so give us falsely elevated and depressed peaks and troughs in our output display. This is the practical example of under-damping, when the arterial pressure is inappropriately over-represented.

At the beginning of the section on damping, we said that it was caused by friction in the measurement system. Using the example of being on the swing again, if you become frightened that your friend is pushing you too hard, and you are swinging too high, what do you do? You scrape your feet along the ground, increasing friction, dissipating energy and therefore reducing the amplitude of your oscillations.

The things that increase damping in our invasive BP monitoring system have been listed above. As users of the system, we cannot actually affect the natural frequency of the system. The only thing we can do theoretically is alter the length of the saline column, but even this is predetermined by the length of the tubing in the 'arterial line' packs. Increasing the length of the saline column will add to damping which you would think would be helpful given that we are worried about augmenting the system's natural oscillations. However, this will decrease the system's natural frequency to a more significant degree and so we tend to move towards an under-damped system, the longer the saline column.

CHAPTER 50

Gas laws

As with most physics questions, the examiner is likely to start by asking you for definitions before trying to make the subject matter clinically relevant.

What is a gas?
A gas is a substance that exists above its critical temperature. This term is usually used colloquially to describe a substance whose critical temperature is below room temperature.

What is critical temperature (CT)?
This is the temperature above which a gas cannot be liquefied by the application of pressure alone (CT for O_2 is $-119°C$ and N_2O is $36.5°C$).

What is an 'ideal gas'?
An 'ideal gas' is a theoretical gas in which the molecules behave as individual particles that move in a random fashion independent of each other and of any inter-molecular forces. At standard temperature and pressure (STP: 273.15 K and 101.3 kPa) most gases behave qualitatively like an ideal gas. The 'ideal gas' is a useful concept because it obeys the ideal gas laws.

What are the gas laws?
The gas laws are a set of rules which govern the relationship between thermodynamic temperature, volume and pressure of ideal gases.
➤ **Boyle's law:** At a constant temperature, the absolute pressure of a given mass of gas is inversely proportional to the volume.

(density = mass/volume → density $\propto$ 1/volume → pressure $\propto$ density)

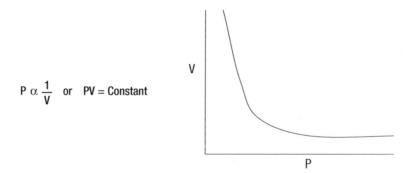

$P \propto \dfrac{1}{V}$ or   PV = Constant

GRAPH 2.7 Boyle's law

➤ **Charles's law:** At a constant pressure, the volume of a given mass of gas is directly proportional to the absolute temperature.

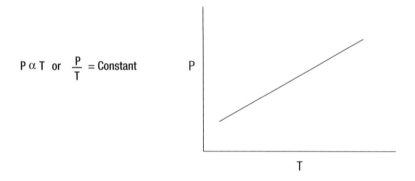

$$V \alpha T \quad \text{or} \quad \frac{V}{T} = \text{Constant}$$

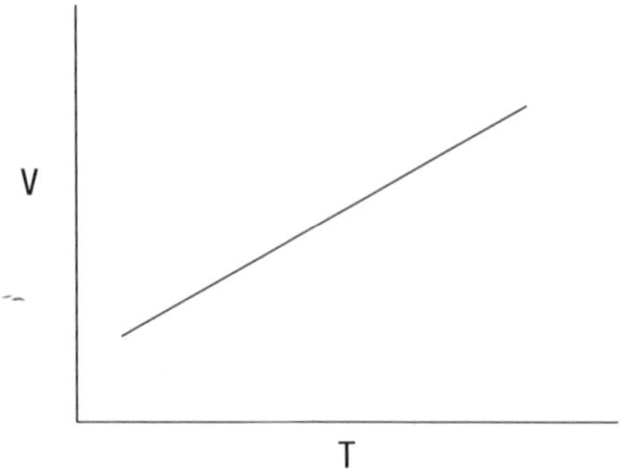

GRAPH 2.8 Charles's law

➤ **Gay-Lussac's law:** At a constant volume, the absolute pressure of a given mass of gas varies directly with the absolute temperature. This is also known as the third perfect gas law.

$$P \alpha T \quad \text{or} \quad \frac{P}{T} = \text{Constant}$$

GRAPH 2.9 Gay-Lussac's law

➤ All of these laws have been united into one, **the Ideal Gas Equation**, which comes from the premise that in an ideal gas, a given number of particles will occupy the same volume at a given temperature and pressure.

$$\frac{PV}{T} = \text{Constant}$$

➤ Using this equation it is possible to convert one set of conditions to another because for a given mass of gas:

$$\frac{P_1 V_1}{T_1} = \frac{P_2 V_2}{T_2}$$

➤ The ideal gas equation is usually written as:

$$PV = nRT$$

Where:
n = number of moles of gas present
R = universal gas constant = $8.32\,J/°C$ at $0°C$ and 1 atmosphere.

What is Avogadro's hypothesis?
This states that equal volumes of gases at a given temperature and pressure contain the same numbers of molecules.

One mole of a gas at STP will occupy 22.4 L and will contain 6.022×10^{23} particles (Avogadro's number).

What is Avogadro's number?
One mole of a substance contains the same number of particles as there are atoms in 12 g of carbon–12 (i.e. 6.022×10^{23}). This number of particles is known as Avogadro's number.

Give an example where we may use Avogadro's hypothesis
Avogadro's hypothesis is used to calculate the contents of a N_2O cylinder:

$$\text{No. of moles of } N_2O \text{ in cylinder} = \text{Weight of } N_2O/\text{Molecular weight of } N_2O$$
$$= (\text{Cylinder weight} - \text{Tare weight})/44$$
$$\text{Volume of } N_2O \text{ available (L)} = \text{No. of moles} \times 22.4 \text{ L}$$

What are the clinical applications of these gas laws?
The ideal gas law $(P_1V_1/T_1 = P_2V_2/T_2)$ is used to calculate the volume of O_2 available from an O_2 cylinder:
➤ Cylinder capacity is fixed = 10 L $[V_1]$
➤ Gauge pressure of cylinder = 13 700 kPa
➤ Absolute pressure of cylinder = gauge pressure (13 700 kPa) + atmospheric pressure (100 kPa) = 13 800 kPa $[P_1]$
➤ Volume of O_2 available = $[V_2]$
➤ Absolute pressure of atmosphere = 100 kPa $[P_2]$
➤ As temperature is constant, $T_1 = T_2$ and hence equation is further simplified

$$P_1 \times V_1 = P_2 \times V_2 \rightarrow 13\,800 \times 10 = 100 \times V_2 \rightarrow V_2 = 1380 \text{ L}$$

➤ But 10 L will always remain in the cylinder and hence 1370 L of O_2 is available.

An alternative approach to this is to use the ideal gas law $(PV/T = nRT)$ to calculate the contents of a gas cylinder:
➤ Volume of the cylinder is fixed
➤ R is a constant
➤ Temperature is fixed
➤ Therefore pressure is directly related to the number of moles of gas (which can be converted into a volume using Avogadro's hypothesis).

The ideal gas law is used in the adiabatic process. If heat energy is not added to or lost from a system, a rapid compression of gas will result in a rise in its temperature, and conversely a sudden expansion will result in a fall. This principle is harnessed by the cryotherapy probe used to freeze lesions in surgery where a sudden expansion of gas through the end leaves its tip extremely cold.

What is Dalton's law of partial pressures?
This states that the total pressure exerted by a gaseous mixture is equal to the sum of the partial pressures of each of the individual gases within that mixture.

What is Henry's law?
This states that the amount of gas dissolved in a liquid is proportional to its partial pressure above that liquid at a given temperature (the warmer the liquid, the less gas that dissolves in it, and that is why boiling water bubbles because air comes out of the liquid phase).

CHAPTER 51

Supply of medical gases

How is oxygen manufactured?
➤ The most common method of manufacturing oxygen commercially is by the fractional distillation of liquefied air. This method produces oxygen which is over 99% pure.
➤ Alternatively, oxygen concentrators containing zeolite adsorbants can be used. Zeolite selectively adsorbs nitrogen and so delivers oxygen that is 90–93% pure. The major contaminant is argon. Oxygen concentrators are commonly used in aircraft, submarines, military field hospitals and at home.

How is oxygen stored?
➤ The main hospital supply of oxygen comes from a vacuum insulated evaporator (VIE), which holds up to 1500 L of liquid oxygen. This is the most economical and space-saving way of storing oxygen. The liquid oxygen is stored at a temperature between −150 and −170°C (below its critical temperature of −119°C) and at a pressure of 7 bar (this is the saturated vapour pressure (SVP) of oxygen at its stored temperature). Because it is in liquid form, oxygen in a VIE behaves like nitrous oxide in a cylinder and therefore in order to know how much oxygen is remaining, the storage vessel rests on a weighing balance so that the mass of liquid oxygen can be measured.
➤ The hospital back-up oxygen supply comes from a cylinder manifold (size J cylinders arranged in series), which stores oxygen as a compressed gas at room temperature. The oxygen from these sites gets carried to the hospital in pipelines coloured white delivered at a pressure of 4 bar (400 kPa).
➤ Oxygen on the anaesthetic machine is stored as a compressed gas in molybdenum steel cylinders (size E cylinders) with black bodies and white shoulders at a pressure of 137 bar (13 700 kPa).

Why are oxygen cylinders filled to 137 bar?
Cylinder technology is old and filling pressures of compressed gases were originally measured is pounds per square inch (psi). The cylinders were filled to 2000 psi, which is equivalent to 137 bar.

How do you calculate the volume of oxygen that can be discharged from a 10 L cylinder?
Oxygen in a cylinder is stored as a compressed gas and obeys the ideal gas law ($P_1V_1/T_1 = P_2V_2/T_2$), which is used to calculate the volume of O_2 available:
➤ Cylinder capacity is fixed = 10 L [V_1]
➤ Gauge pressure of cylinder = 13 700 kPa
➤ Absolute pressure of cylinder = gauge pressure (13 700 kPa) + atmospheric pressure (100 kPa) = 13 800 kPa [P_1]
➤ Volume of O_2 available = [V_2]
➤ Pressure of atmosphere = 100 kPa [P_2]
➤ As temperature is constant, $T_1 = T_2$ and hence equation is further simplified

$$P_1 \times V_1 = P_2 \times V_2 \rightarrow 13\,800 \times 10 = 100 \times V_2 \rightarrow V_2 = 1380\,L$$

➤ But 10 L will always remain in the cylinder and hence 1370 L of O_2 is available.

Draw a graph showing what would happen to the gauge pressure of an oxygen cylinder over time if it were being used continuously at the same rate

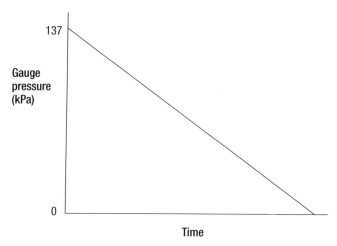

GRAPH 2.10 Change in gauge pressure over time for an O_2 cylinder

How is nitrous oxide manufactured?
Nitrous oxide (N_2O) is manufactured by the thermal decomposition of ammonium nitrate.

How is nitrous oxide stored?
➤ The critical temperature of nitrous oxide is 36.5°C and therefore at room temperature N_2O exists as a liquid with its vapour.
➤ On the anaesthetic machine, N_2O is stored as a liquid in molybdenum steel cylinders with blue bodies and blue shoulders at a pressure of 52 bar (this is the SVP of N_2O vapour above its liquid).
➤ N_2O cylinders are only partially filled because liquids are less compressible than gases and should these cylinders be subjected to temperatures above its critical temperature (e.g. in a desert or during a fire) all the N_2O would convert to a gas causing a massive explosion. Therefore, depending on the temperature of the country, N_2O cylinders have different filling ratios.

The filling ratio = $\dfrac{\text{Weight of substance cylinder is routinely filled with}}{\text{Weight of water cylinder could hold if full}}$

➤ In tropical countries the filling ratio is 0.67 but in temperate climates it is 0.75.
➤ The main hospital supply of N_2O comes from a cylinder manifold where once again the N_2O is stored as a liquid at room temperature.

Why do different textbooks quote varying gauge pressures for N_2O cylinders?
N_2O cylinder gauge pressures reflect the SVP of the N_2O above its liquid and are quoted from between 44 bar to 54 bar depending on the temperature at which the measurement was taken (as SVP varies with temperature).

How can you calculate the volume of N_2O that can be discharged from a cylinder? Because these cylinders contain liquid and vapour you cannot apply the ideal gas law. Instead you need to weigh the cylinder in order to work out the weight of the remaining N_2O and then apply Avogadro's hypothesis:

> **No. of moles of N_2O in cylinder = Weight of N_2O/Molecular weight of N_2O**
> **= (Cylinder weight – Tare weight)/44**
> **Volume of N_2O available (L) = No. of moles × 22.4 L**

Avogadro's hypothesis states that at standard temperature and pressure 1 mole of gas occupies 22.4 L.

Draw a graph showing what would happen to the gauge pressure of a nitrous oxide cylinder over time if it were being used continuously at the same rate

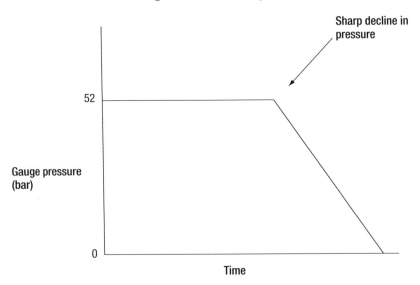

GRAPH 2.11 Change in gauge pressure over time for a N_2O cylinder

➤ Initially, the N_2O cylinder contains both liquid and vapour.
➤ As the cylinder empties, the vapour is used up and the liquid continues to vaporise until it is all used up.
➤ This explains the constant cylinder gauge pressure until all the liquid has been used up, at which point the cylinder only contains gas and behaves like the oxygen cylinder and obeys Boyle's law, with pressure declining over time with use.
➤ This is actually a simplification; in reality the initial pressure is not perfectly constant because as the N_2O vaporises from the liquid phase it cools slightly (latent heat of vaporisation), and therefore gauge pressure does fall slightly.

Define the following terms
➤ **Gas** – exists in the gaseous state because at room temperature it is above its critical temperature (and therefore cannot be liquefied by the application of pressure).
➤ **Vapour** – gaseous state of a substance which at room temperature exists normally as a liquid because it is below its critical temperature.
➤ **Critical temperature** – temperature above which a substance cannot be liquefied no matter how much pressure is applied.

➤ **Pseudocritical temperature** – applies to a mixture of gases (e.g. entonox – 50% O_2 and 50% N_2O) and is the temperature at which these gases may separate out into their individual constituents.

➤ **Critical pressure** – pressure required to liquefy a gas at its critical temperature.

What is the Poynting effect?

If a gas mixture is exposed to a temperature below its pseudocritical temperature the individual gas components can liquefy and separate out. This is known as the Poynting effect and is important in relation to entonox cylinders. If entonox cylinders are allowed to fall below –5.5°C (e.g. during mountain rescues) a liquid mixture containing mostly N_2O with only about 20% O_2 dissolved in it can form along with a high oxygen content gas mixture just above it. If this cylinder is then used, the patient will initially receive an O_2 rich gas mixture but as the cylinder is used up the O_2 concentration will progressively decrease and eventually the patient may receive a hypoxic gas mixture. In order to minimise these risks, entonox cylinders should be stored horizontally at temperatures above 5°C.

TABLE 2.12 Key features of commonly used medical gases

Content	State	Cylinder colour (cylinder/shoulder)	Cylinder pressure (bar)	Critical temperature (°C)
Oxygen	Gas	Black/White	137	–119
Nitrous oxide	Vapour	Blue/Blue	52	36.5
Air	Gas	Black/Black & White	137	–141
Carbon dioxide	Vapour	Grey/Grey	50	31
Entonox	Gas mix	Blue/Blue & White	137	–5.5 (pseudocritical)
Heliox	Gas	Brown/Brown & White	137	

CHAPTER 52

General aspects of pressure

'Dum dum dum didi da dum insanity laughs under pressure we're cracking'

—David Bowie

Questions on pressure can start innocently enough but can lead to almost any aspect of anaesthesia. One college question starts by comparing the pressure generated in 2 mL and 20 mL syringes and ends up with altitude effects via calibration of pressure transducers.

Define pressure
Pressure is the force applied per unit area. Its SI unit is the pascal (N/m^2).

What is force?
Force is a vector quantity that can cause an object with mass to accelerate. Newton's second law defined force as the mass of an object multiplied by it acceleration. Its SI unit is the newton.

One newton will accelerate a 1 kg mass at $1 m/s^2$ in a vacuum. Gravity gives any object an acceleration of $9.81 m/s^2$ making one newton equivalent to a 102 g weight. This is a small pressure when applied to a squared metre area, so pressure is normally expressed in kilopascals (kPa).

What other units of pressure are there?
1 bar is equivalent to:
➤ 1 atmosphere
➤ 14.5 lb/in^2 (psi)
➤ 30 inches of Hg
➤ 101 kPa
➤ 760 mmHg (torr)
➤ 1020 cmH$_2$O

Are you more likely to dislodge a blockage in the nozzle of a syringe when using a 2 mL or 20 mL syringe?
A 2 mL syringe, as pressure is force over area. The 2 mL syringe has a smaller cross-sectional area so the force applied by the thumb is spread over a smaller area generating a higher pressure. For this reason care must be taken when injecting fluids with a small syringe as the high pressure generated could cause tissue damage.

What is the difference between partial and total pressures?
Dalton's law states that in a gas mixture the pressure exerted by each individual gas is equal to the pressure that gas would exert if it alone occupied the container. This is the partial pressure (the term 'tension' refers to the pressure exerted by a gas dissolved in liquid).

Total pressure is the sum of all the partial pressures in the mixture.

Is atmospheric pressure constant?

No. Atmospheric pressure is created by the force of gravity acting on the molecules that make up the atmosphere and therefore atmospheric pressure will depend on the height of the atmosphere and its density. This means that atmospheric pressure will fall with altitude and rising temperature. As a consequence, the partial pressure of the gases that make up the air will also fall, leading to low partial pressures of oxygen at altitude.

What is gauge pressure?

Gauge pressure refers to pressure measurements above or below atmospheric pressure. An empty cylinder pressure will have a gauge pressure of zero.

What is absolute pressure?

Absolute pressure refers to pressure measurements incorporating atmospheric pressure – it is gauge pressure plus atmospheric pressure. An empty cylinder will have an absolute pressure of 1 bar.

Is blood pressure an absolute or gauge pressure?

Blood pressure is a gauge pressure.

How do manometers work?

➤ A manometer consists of a fluid-filled column, which is open to the atmosphere and therefore reads gauge pressure.
➤ Gravity acts on the fluid to produce a pressure, which is dependent on the density of the fluid and the height of the fluid but independent of the cross-sectional area of the column (pressure = height × density × gravitational force).
➤ They are used to measure low pressures.
➤ Inaccuracies can be caused by surface tension. This leads to an over-reading in water manometers and an under-reading in mercury manometers (in practice this has no clinical significance as a 6 mm wide column of water will only over-read by 0.04 kPa).
➤ They can be made more sensitive by using fluids with a low density (e.g. a pressure of 1 kPa will support a column of mercury 7.5 mm high or a column of water 10.2 cm high).

What are barometers?

➤ Barometers are closed to the atmosphere and therefore measure absolute pressure.
➤ A mercury barometer has a torricellian vacuum above it, which contains mercury vapour at its SVP.
➤ Barometers like the Fortin's barometer and Goethe's device can be used to measure sub-atmospheric pressures. Here the height of the measuring column falls rather than rises and this principle was used to predict bad weather; low atmospheric pressures would cause a fall in the height of the fluid in a 'thunder tube', predicting an oncoming storm.

How do aneroid gauges work?

➤ Aneroid gauges (from the Greek meaning 'no water') such as the Bourdon gauge are used to measure high pressures where manometers would be impractical (e.g. to measure the pressure of a 137 bar oxygen cylinder you would need a mercury column 104 m high or a water column 1394 m high!).
➤ A Bourdon gauge consists of a coiled metal tube linked to a cog and a pointer. The cross-sectional area of the tube is elliptical and when exposed to increases in pressure it changes to a circular cross-sectional shape, which causes the tube to uncoil, moving the pointer across a scale.

CHAPTER 53

Pressure regulators

Questions about pressure regulators are likely to start with simple quick questions about the different pressures that gases are stored and delivered at and then move on to how these changes in pressure are achieved.

What are the pressures at which the common anaesthetic gases are stored and delivered at?

TABLE 2.13 Storage and delivery pressures for commonly used medical gases

Site	Oxygen	Air	Nitrous oxide
Cylinder pressure	137 bar	137 bar	52 bar (room temp.)
Pipeline pressure	4 bar	4 bar	4 bar
Common gas outlet pressure	2 cmH$_2$O	2 cmH$_2$O	2 cmH$_2$O

Define the following terms

Pressure – force per unit area. The SI unit is the pascal (N/m^2). Other commonly used units are the kilopascal, mmHg, cmH$_2$0, psi, bar, torr and atm (*see* question on 'General aspects of pressure').

Pressure regulators (or pressure-reducing valves) – devices that reduce a higher variable inlet pressure to a constant lower outlet pressure.

What different types of pressure regulators do you know?
The different types of pressure regulators may be classified as follows:
➤ **Direct** – where the cylinder pressure opens the valve
➤ **Indirect** – where a spring opens the valve in response to falling outlet pressure
➤ **Two-stage** – where the input of one is the output of the other, this reduces wear on the diaphragm and reduces pressure fluctuations in high gas flows (e.g. demand valves used on entonox cylinders)
➤ **Slave** – where the output of one valve is dependent on the output of another (e.g. nitrous oxide valve will not open unless there is output from the O$_2$ valve).

Why is the gas cylinder on an anaesthetic machine not connected directly to the rotameter block?
Gas (and vapour) cylinders are used to store gases and vapours at high pressures. These pressures vary according to the type of gas or vapour used, the cylinder content and temperature. The temperature and cylinder content will in turn vary as the gas or vapour is used. If unregulated this would lead to a variable flow of gas or vapour to the patient. In order to provide a safe and constant mixture of gases during anaesthesia it is important to protect both the patient and anaesthetic machine from exposure to higher pressures, surges in pressure when cylinders are opened and changes in flow. This is achieved by using pressure regulators, flow

restrictors and pressure relief valves. It is important to note that the pressure regulators are specific to particular gases and are set during servicing.

How does a single stage regulator work?
➤ Pressure regulators consist of two chambers, a high pressure chamber and a low or control pressure chamber, separated by a conical valve whose orifice is controlled by a spring connected to a diaphragm in the control chamber.
➤ They work by balancing the force from the spring against the force generated by pressure against the diaphragm.
➤ The relationship between the force from the spring and the pressures in the two chambers is given by:

$$F = Pa + pA$$

Where:

F	is the force from the spring (adjustable)
P	is the high inlet pressure
a	is the area of valve
p	is the low outlet pressure
A	is the area of the diaphragm

➤ This shows that the performance of the valve is related to the ratio of the areas of the diaphragm and the valve: the bigger the difference the greater the drop in pressure for the same force applied by the spring.

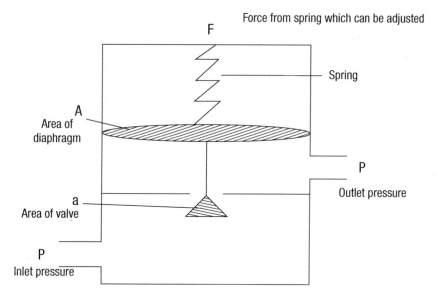

FIGURE 2.14 Single-staged pressure regulator

➤ From the diagram it can be seen that if the inlet pressure (P) increases the diaphragm will lift and the conical valve will shut and vice versa. The pressure in the control chamber can be fixed or varied by altering the tension in the spring.

How does a two-stage pressure regulator work?
➤ A demand valve on an entonox cylinder or diving cylinder is an example of a two-stage pressure regulator.

➤ The 1st stage of the regulator is identical to that already described but now the flow of gas from the low-pressure chamber enters the 2nd stage chamber.
➤ The 2nd stage chamber contains a larger diaphragm that operates a valve, which connects it to the 1st stage low-pressure chamber.
➤ The demand valve detects when the patient inspires and supplies them with a breath of gas at ambient pressure.
➤ As the patient inspires, the pressure within the 2nd stage chamber reduces, moving the diaphragm, which opens the valve and allows gas to enter the 2nd stage chamber from the 1st stage low-pressure chamber.

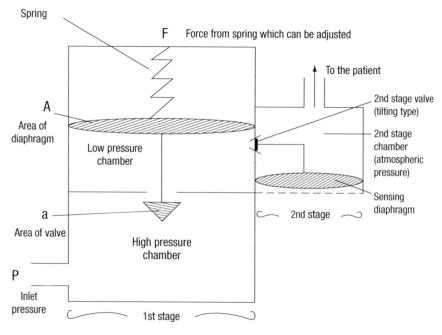

FIGURE 2.15 Two-stage demand valve

How does the Ritchie whistle work?
➤ The Ritchie whistle is an oxygen failure alarm, which is powered solely by falling oxygen pressures.
➤ It was invented by John Ritchie, a New Zealand anaesthetist, and was introduced into practice in the mid-1960s.
➤ Again, its design was tailored around a single-stage pressure regulator.
➤ Its working principle is simple: as the oxygen pressure falls, the force acting on the diaphragm reduces and a point is reached when the opposing force applied by the spring is greater, allowing the valve to open and oxygen to leak past and activate the whistle.
➤ Current oxygen failure devices must have an auditory sound of at least 60 dB lasting for 7 s and should be activated when oxygen pressure falls to 200 kPa. It should be linked to a system that shuts off the supply of all other gases apart from oxygen and air.
➤ Modern devices now use electronic sensors.

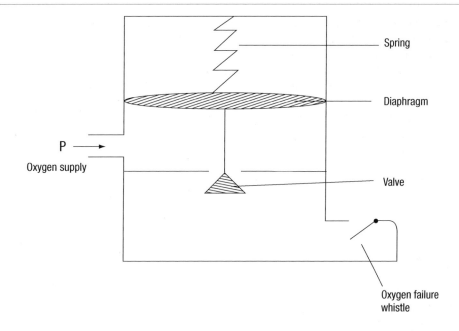

P $\longrightarrow$

Oxygen supply

Spring

Diaphragm

Valve

Oxygen failure
whistle

FIGURE 2.16 Ritchie whistle

CHAPTER 54

Flow

There are many aspects of flow that are of particular relevance to anaesthetic practice and thus examination questions may take various directions. However, the fundamental principles regarding flow are the same irrespective of the application.

What is flow?
Flow is the quantity of a fluid passing a point per unit time.

What are the characteristics of laminar flow?
➤ Fluid moves in a steady manner (no eddies or turbulence).
➤ Flow rate is greatest at the centre of the flow stream (2 × flow rate at side of tube).
➤ A pressure difference must exist for fluid to flow.
➤ Flow is directly proportional to this pressure difference.
➤ Resistance of the tube is calculated by the ratio of pressure to flow.

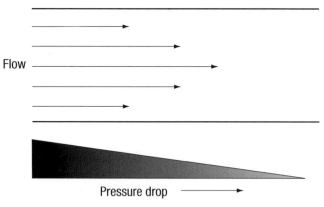

FIGURE 2.17 Laminar flow

What equation can be used to calculate laminar flow?
Hagen-Poiseuille equation is used to calculate laminar flow:

$$\text{Flow} = \frac{\pi \times \Delta P \times r^4}{8 \times L \times n}$$

Where:
π = Pi (mathematical constant – the ratio of any circle's circumference to its diameter)
ΔP = Pressure drop
r = Radius
L = Length of tube
n = Viscosity of fluid

Thus:
➤ Flow is proportional to the pressure drop and radius of the tube.
➤ Flow is inversely proportional to the length of tube and the viscosity of the fluid.

Give an example where the Hagen-Poiseuille equation is clinically applied
Administering a unit of blood rapidly to a patient:
➤ Use a short, wide-bore cannula.
➤ Raise the height of the giving set.
➤ Apply a pressure bag to the unit of blood.
➤ Warm the blood pre-administration (reduces viscosity).

What are the characteristics of turbulent flow?
➤ Flow characterised by swirls and eddies.
➤ Transition of laminar to turbulent flow may occur at constrictions.
➤ Fluid velocity varies across the tube.
➤ Flow is proportional to the square root of pressure (i.e. to double flow, the pressure
   must be increased by a factor of 4).
➤ Resistance is no longer constant because the relationship between pressure and flow is
   no longer linear.
➤ Density of the fluid is the important determinant in turbulent flow (as opposed to
   fluid viscosity in laminar flow).

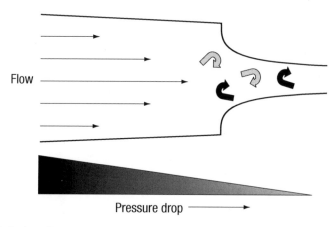

FIGURE 2.18 Turbulent flow

Thus:
➤ Flow is proportional to the square root of pressure.
➤ Flow is proportional to the radius squared.
➤ Flow is inversely proportional to the square root of the tube length.
➤ Flow is inversely proportional to the square root of fluid density.

What is Reynolds number?
This is a number that predicts the onset of turbulent flow of a fluid:

$$\text{Reynolds number} = \frac{\text{Velocity of fluid} \times \text{Density} \times \text{Tube diameter}}{\text{Viscosity}}$$

➤ Reynolds number < 2000 predicts laminar flow
➤ Reynolds number > 2000 predicts turbulent flow

Give an example where the concept of Reynolds number is used clinically
The use of helium in upper airway obstruction – helium reduces the density of inhaled gas, thereby lowering the Reynolds number, which results in a change of flow from turbulent to laminar. Laminar flow is known to reduce the work of breathing.

What is the critical velocity?
This is the velocity above which the flow of a fluid within a given tube is likely to change from laminar to turbulent (e.g. critical velocity of gas flow in a 9 mm endotracheal tube is 9 L/min).

What is the Bernoulli effect?
Bernoulli effect refers to a fall in pressure at a constriction in a tube. At the constriction point, the kinetic energy of a fluid increases and by the 'law of conservation of energy' this means that the pressure at this point must fall in order for total energy to remain constant.

What is the Venturi principle?
This utilises the Bernoulli effect to entrain a second fluid at the point of low pressure. The **entrainment ratio** describes the ratio of entrained flow to driving flow. Venturi oxygen delivery masks, nebulisers and suction devices provide good clinical examples.

What is the Coanda effect?
This is the tendency of a fluid jet to stay attached to an adjacent curved surface. The principle was named after Henry Coandă, who was the first to recognise the practical application of the phenomenon in the development of jet engines. This tendency of fluid flow to not divide evenly explains the maldistribution of gas flow to alveoli where there has been a slight narrowing of the bronchiole before it divides.

How can flow be measured?
➤ **Wright respirometer:** This device actually measures gas volumes but flow can be calculated by measuring the volume of gas per unit time.
  ● Device used to measure tidal volumes in anaesthesia
  ● Gas flow rotates vanes
  ● Inaccurate for continuous flow
  ● Over-reads at high flow rates
  ● Under-reads at low flow rates
➤ **Pneumotachograph:** A constant orifice, variable pressure device used to measure flow. Flow is calculated by measuring the pressure difference across a fixed orifice.
  ● Device used to measure gas flow.
  ● A constant orifice, variable pressure device.
  ● Gauze screen acts as a resistance to flow and maintains laminar flow.
  ● Airflow causes a pressure drop across the gauze screen, which is measured by a pressure transducer and correlates with flow.
  ● Pressure difference across the gauze is proportional flow (provided flow is laminar).
  ● Pressure change is converted into an electrical signal and displayed.
➤ **Rotameters:** A constant pressure, variable orifice device used in anaesthetic machines to act as a continuous indicator of gas flows.
  ● Device used to measure gas flow.
  ● Constant pressure, variable orifice device.
  ● Bobbin in a tapered glass tube.
  ● Rotating bobbin rises as flow increases.
  ● Pressure across the bobbin remains constant.

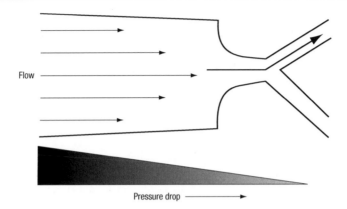

FIGURE 2.19 Flow at a constriction

- Mixture of laminar and turbulent flow exists, therefore for calibration purposes, both the viscosity and density of the fluid are important.
- Electrostatic charges can develop around the bobbin, which is minimised by the incorporation of a conductive strip.

CHAPTER 55

Electrical components

Questions on electrical components are often asked as part of a question on defibrillators (*see* Chapter 56 on 'Defibrillators'). Typically, a card with various electrical symbols will be shown to the candidate and this will lead on to questions regarding the various components. Another favourite topic is amplification and the Wheatstone bridge including the concept of null deflection, so it is worth spending the time to understand how these work.

Explain the following terms
➤ **Resistance:**
  - Opposition to flow of direct current.
  - It is represented by the symbols R and its unit is the ohm (Ω).
  - $1\,\Omega$ is the resistance that will allow 1 A of current to flow when a potential of 1 V is applied across it.
  - The resistance of different electrical components can vary with physical stresses such as temperature and stretch. These changes are exploited in electrical thermometers and transducers.
  - Resistance is key to Ohm's law ($V = I \times R$), which is a fundamental equation in electronics.
➤ **Reactance:**
  - Opposition to the flow of alternating current caused by the inductance and capacitance in a circuit rather than by resistance.
  - It decreases with increasing current frequency.
  - It is represented by the symbol X and its unit is the Ω.
➤ **Impedance:**
  - Total opposition to current flow in an alternating current circuit, made up of two components, resistance and reactance.
  - It is represented by the symbol Z and its unit is the Ω.
➤ **Capacitor:**
  - Device that can store charge.
  - It consists of two conducting plates separated by an insulator (dielectric).
  - The amount of charge that it can store depends on the size of the plates, separation gap and the dielectric material.
  - It blocks DC (high resistance) but passes AC (low reactance) as the plates get alternately charged and discharged.
  - As reactance decreases with increasing current frequency, diathermy devices with high frequencies of 1.5 MHz will have low reactance and hence will be conducted. Mains electricity at 50 Hz has a high reactance and therefore will not be conducted. This property makes capacitors useful filters.
  - Also its stored energy can be rapidly discharged, making it the central component of the defibrillator.
  - Charge (Q) is measured in coulombs (C), 1 C being the number of electrons passing a point when a current of 1 A flows for 1 s (6.24×10^{18} electrons).

- Capacitance (C) is measured in farads (F), 1 F being the capacity to hold 1 C of charge when a potential difference of 1 V is applied.
- The energy stored by a capacitor is given by the formula $E = \frac{1}{2}QV$ or $E = \frac{1}{2}CV^2$.

➤ **Inductor:**
- Device that 'induces' a magnetic field.
- It consists of a wire coiled around a ferrous core (former).
- As current flows through the coiled wire a magnetic field is generated.
- These block AC (high reactance) but pass DC (low resistance).
- These are a source of interference in electrical equipment where electromotive activity in one circuit can induce unwanted signals in another.
- They are used in transformers and to isolate equipment from earth (floating circuits – see Chapter 57, 'Electrical safety') and are also used in defibrillators to smoothen and lengthen the current pulse.

➤ **Transformer:**
- Transform voltages up or down (step up or step down).
- Consist of two inductors wound around the same former (core). This close relationship means that current changes in one circuit can induce current in the second circuit due to the coupling effects of the magnetic field.
- They are used to step up the voltage of a current to allow efficient transmission over large distances and to step the voltage down to levels suitable for household use.
- They are also used as isolating transformers (see Chapter 57) where they isolate appliances from earth.
- The change in voltage from the primary circuit to the secondary circuit is calculated from Faraday's law of induction, where the ratio of the number of coils of each circuit around the transformer core determines whether there is an increase or decrease in the voltage from one to the other.

➤ **Earth:**
- System of electrical safety where there is an electrical connection to ground.
- This protects people from the effects of faulty insulation in electrically powered equipment, as there is significantly less resistance through the earth circuit than there is through the person.
- Class 1 equipment is earthed (see Chapter 57).

➤ **Diode (or rectifier):**
- Allows current to flow in one direction only.

➤ **Battery (or voltaic cell):**
- Collection of galvanic cells that store chemical energy and can release it as electrical energy when part of an electrical circuit.
- They consist of two half-cells (negative cathode and positive cathode) connected by a conductive electrolyte.
- Oxidation occurs at the anode and reduction at the cathode, allowing a flow of electrons between the two.

➤ **Transducer:**
- Changes one form of energy into another, normally into an electronic signal for interpretation and recording.
- Examples include the microphone, which converts sound energy into an electrical signal, and the pressure transducer, which converts pressure changes into electrical resistance.

➤ **Amplifier:**

- Differs from a transducer in that it makes the input signal larger for easier interpretation rather than changing it from one form to another.
- They are used because biological signals are often very small (EEG signals in the order of micro-volts) and need to be made bigger (amplified) for display.
- Amplifiers do not need to be electrical. Levers can produce a large movement at one end of a needle from a small movement at the other (Bourdon gauge) and microscopes convert a small light field into a large one.
- For electrical signals, amplifiers increase the amplitude of the signal.
- The difference in the size of the input signal and the amplified signal is called the gain and is measured in bels (or decibels).
- In the amplification process there will inevitably be an amplification of unwanted signal. This is called the noise. The amount of noise introduced compared to the signal is called the signal to noise ratio and is a measure of the performance of the system.
- To reduce the amount of noise, amplifiers can also act as filters. They can achieve this in a number of ways. Firstly, amplifiers are often differential amplifiers (also called operational amplifiers), that is, they look for signals that vary from one source to another (e.g. different leads on an ECG) and amplify them, rejecting signals that are common to both as interference. This is called common mode rejection. If we consider the ECG signal again, the R wave will differ from lead to lead so will be amplified for the ECG trace. However, 50 Hz mains interference will be the same at all leads and so will be rejected. They also have the advantage of being high-gain amplifiers without the need for additional power. Amplifiers also filter by amplifying only a certain frequency range (bandwidth filter), signals above or below a certain frequency (high or low pass filters), rejecting particular frequencies (notch filter, e.g. 50 Hz mains signal) and by amplifying signals of a particular amplitude.

CHAPTER 56

Defibrillators

Defibrillators are devices used to restore normal cardiac rhythm by delivering electrical energy to the heart, which causes co-ordinated myocardial depolarisation. There are various types that can be manual or automated, monophasic or biphasic, external, transvenous or implanted in the patient.

What is the difference between monophasic and biphasic waveform defibrillators?
➤ **Monophasic waveform:** This is a dampened sinusoidal wave (Lown-type waveform). Current flows in one direction only, from one electrode to the other.
➤ **Biphasic waveform:** This can be either a biphasic truncated exponential waveform or a rectilinear biphasic waveform. Current flows in alternating directions, completing one cycle in approximately 10 ms. During the first phase current flows in one direction and then reverses direction during the second phase. This lowers the electrical threshold for successful defibrillation allowing lower energy levels to be used, which reduces the risk of burns and myocardial damage. Biphasic defibrillation was originally developed and used for implantable cardioverter defibrillators.

Draw the major components in a defibrillator circuit

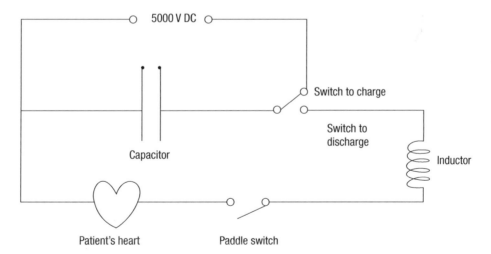

FIGURE 2.20 Components of a defibrillator circuit

How does a defibrillator work?
➤ Delivers DC shock instead of AC (less myocardial damage and less arrythmogenic).
➤ Uses 5000 V (this is much greater than that of the mains electricity and is produced using a step-up transformer).
➤ Capacitor is used to store charge. It consists of two conducting plates separated by an insulating material (dielectric). Capacitance is measured in farads (F). The amount

of charge it can store depends on the size of the plates, their separating gap and the dielectric material. They have a low reactance to AC (i.e. passes AC) but a high resistance to DC (i.e. blocks DC).

Charge (Q) = Capacitance (C) × Voltage (V)
Energy stored (E) = ½ CV²

➤ Inductor is used to prolong the duration of current discharge. It consists of coils of conducting material wound around a ferrous core (former). A magnetic flux is induced whenever a current flows through the coils. They have a high reactance to AC (i.e. block AC) but a low resistance to DC (i.e. pass DC).
➤ Produces a DC shock from 30 A, for 3 ms with 5000 V.
➤ Delivered (quoted) energy is less than stored charge due to some loss within the inductor.
➤ Thoracic impedance is in the region of 50–150 Ω and this is reduced after the first shock, by the use of conductive gel pads, front-to-back defibrillation and application of firm paddle pressure.
➤ Internal defibrillators use 20–50 J, biphasic use 150 J and monophasic use 360 J.
➤ During cardioversion, a synchronised DC shock must be administered in order to prevent 'R on T' phenomenon, which can trigger VF.
➤ During defibrillation of pulseless VT or VF, a non-synchronised shock can be administered.

How can you calculate the energy that will be delivered during a shock?
This can be done using the equation E = ½ CV²
➤ If C is 100 μF and V is 2000 V
➤ Then E = ½ (0.0001)(2000²) = 200 J
➤ Energy stored will be 200 J.

In reality the energy delivered will be slightly less due to some loss within the system.

CHAPTER 57

Electrical safety

Questions on electrical safety do not have many places to go. That being said, it means that you do not have much room for manoeuvre if you do not know about it.

It is important to know about the different forms of electricity, the various circuit set-ups and the specific dangers of each in order to answer a question on safety measures with any confidence. Below are slightly wordier answers than you will have to give but they should cover any selection of questions.

How is mains electricity supplied?
➤ Mains electricity is an alternating current (AC) supplied at 50 Hz and at 240 V.
➤ In AC, the flow of electric charge reverses direction periodically, producing a sine wave pattern.
➤ Electricity is delivered as AC to allow it to be transmitted over large distances (hundreds of miles) with very minimal loss of power. This is in sharp contrast to direct current (DC), which has a dramatic loss of power over just one mile.
➤ AC is generated at a voltage specific to the power plant generator. The voltage is then stepped up (using a transformer) to allow more efficient transfer of power over long distances before being stepped down (using a transformer) to 240 V for use.

What is the significance of the earth wire?
➤ UK mains electricity supply has three wires: live wire (brown), neutral wire (blue) and earth wire (green).
➤ The neutral wire is so called because it is connected to the earth at the mains transformer so its electrical potential is 'neutral' with the earth.
➤ The live and neutral wires are relatively simple to understand but the earth often causes some confusion as on the one hand it is described as a safety measure but on the other hand it is imperative to protect the patient from exposure to earth. This is further complicated by the fact that the earth wire has different names like 'ground', which can mean different things in different circuits.
➤ The earth wire is a safety feature of electrical circuits designed to protect people from exposure to the full current of mains electricity in faulty appliances. It is a wire that literally returns to earth and completes a circuit with the generating power station and is connected to any exposed conducting parts of an electrical appliance.
➤ This means that if the live wire came into contact with a conducting part of the appliance, electricity would flow through it to earth. If the earth was not connected, someone touching the appliance would inadvertently act as a conduit for the electricity to flow and receive a severe shock. By having the earth there, the electricity flows preferentially down the earth wire (because earth is so large and therefore always offers the path of least resistance) rather than through the victim.
➤ Due to the deliberate application of tissue damaging currents (diathermy) patients must be protected from contact with earth. If a patient was inadvertently connected to earth, they would provide an alternative route for the diathermy current to flow

through, which could potentially cause severe burns at the point of contact between the patient and earth. Another safety reason is to prevent the flow of leakage currents from faulty equipment through the patient.

What do the adverse effects of a current depend on?

➤ **Type of current:** AC is significantly more dangerous than DC. AC can cause tetanic muscular contractions ('can't let go' phenomenon) which peak at 50 Hz (frequency of mains electricity). This frequency is also particularly dangerous to the heart, making it prone to VF. With DC, there is a single muscle contraction, which typically throws the victim clear.
➤ **Magnitude of current** (V = I × R)
➤ **Current density** (total current/area)
➤ **Current duration** (increased time means increased heat and hence increased tissue damage)
➤ **Tissues through which current flows** (cardiac muscle is prone to VF).

At what current amplitude would you feel tingling?

➤ 0–5 mA – tingling
➤ 5–10 mA – pain
➤ 10–50 mA – muscle spasm (15 mA 'can't let go' threshold)
➤ 50–100 mA – respiratory muscle spasm and VF
➤ 5 A – tonic contraction of the myocardium (this level of current is rarely seen except in defibrillation).

How can a pair of shoes keep you safe from current?

➤ This is all based on Ohm's law of V= I × R
➤ Resistance of skin is approximately 2000 Ω, body tissue is 500 Ω and shoes are 200 000 Ω.
➤ If a current was to enter skin, pass through body tissues and then exit through skin again, the total resistance it would encounter would be 4500 Ω (2000 + 500 + 2000).
➤ The magnitude of this current would therefore be:

$$I = V/R \rightarrow 240/4500 \rightarrow 53\,mA \text{ (person at risk of arrhythmia)}$$

➤ If current were to enter skin, pass through body tissues and then exit through shoes, the total resistance it would encounter would be 202 500 Ω (2000 + 500 + 200 000).
➤ The magnitude of this current would now be:

$$I = V/R \rightarrow 240/202\,500 \rightarrow 1.2\,mA \text{ (person would feel tingling sensation)}$$

What is a macroshock?

Macroshocks are due to the passage of current from one part of the body to another (e.g. lightning or direct contact with a 'live' instrument whereby the body completes the circuit between the mains and earth). Current intensities required to cause harm are in the region of mA.

What is a microshock?

Microshocks are due to the passage of current directly to the myocardium (e.g. small leakage currents can pass through the heart via central lines, PA catheters and pacing wires). Current intensities required to cause harm are very small in the region of μA.

How is electrical equipment classified?

Electrical equipment is classified by its protection from mains electricity and by its allowable leakage current.

For mains protection it is classified as:

➤ **Class I** – earthed casing (all conducting surfaces are earthed)
➤ **Class II** – double insulated casing (no exposed conducting surface and so does not need to be earthed)
➤ **Class III** – battery-operated

For allowable leakage current it is classified as:

➤ **B** – leakage current up to 0.5 mA, not suitable for surface contact with patient.
➤ **BF** – floating circuit (parts attached to the patient are isolated from the rest of the equipment) with leakage currents up to 0.1 mA, suitable for external contact with patient (e.g. ECG, ultrasound).
➤ **CF** – floating circuit with leakage currents up to 0.01 mA, suitable for contact with the patient's heart (e.g. pulmonary artery floatation catheters).

What other measures are taken in theatre to prevent electrical injury?

➤ **Anti-static flooring** – this has high impedance to mains electricity but enough conductance to earth to prevent the build up of static electricity.
➤ **Relative humidity of 50%** – inhibits the build-up of static electricity.
➤ **Circuit breakers** – these consist of a transformer attached to a solenoid that will break a circuit or sound an alarm if a stray current above a set limit is detected flowing to earth.
➤ **Non-sparking switches and plugs.**
➤ **Regular checks and maintenance of equipment.**

CHAPTER 58

Diathermy

What are the basic principles of diathermy?

➤ Diathermy devices are surgical instruments used to cut tissues and coagulate blood vessels.
➤ They use the heating effect of high frequency AC (0.5–1.0 MHz) passing through tissues of high impedance to burn or vaporise tissues in contact with the diathermy instrument.
➤ The heating effect of a current depends on the current density and duration.
➤ In diathermy the current density at the point where the instrument makes contact with the tissue is very high.
➤ In 'cutting' mode the current flows in an alternating sine wave pattern while in 'coagulation' mode the current flows in a pulsed sine wave pattern.
➤ Diathermy devices can either be monopolar or bipolar.
➤ In monopolar diathermy, current flows through a probe (active electrode) at a high current density and then returns via a diathermy plate (neutral plate) at low current density. The overall power that can be delivered is in the region of 100–400 W.
➤ In bipolar diathermy, the current is passed between two probes within a modified pair of forceps. One probe delivers the current and the second acts as the return circuit so tissues between the probes are exposed to the current and heated. This system helps keep the electrical field focal. The overall power this system can generate is approximately 40 W.

Why is the diathermy pad always checked at the end of surgery?

In bipolar diathermy the current makes a short journey across the tissue and is returned at a similar density, heating all the tissue between the electrodes. In monopolar diathermy the current exits at a point distant from the site of surgery so it is important to ensure that the current density is low enough not to cause injury at this point. Hence the neutral plate has a large surface area and is applied over an area of good blood supply so that the current density is low and any heat generated can be dissipated by the blood flow. If the plate is not applied properly the reduced area or increased impedance can lead to more heat generation and burns, hence the reason the plate site is checked at the end of surgery.

What are the hazards of diathermy?

➤ **Burns:**
  • Incorrect positioning of the neutral plate.
  • Ignition of flammable skin preps.
  • Inadvertent activation of diathermy probe (minimised by audible note when in use and use of a designated holder).
➤ **Electric shocks:**
  • Disconnection of the neutral plate may lead to current passing through an alternative route (e.g. ECG electrodes or exiting through a site where the patient

may be in contact with a conducting surface). This can cause electrical shocks and burns to the patient.

➤ **Pacemaker interference:**
- Ideally, diathermy should be avoided in patients with pacemakers and implantable cardioverter defibrillators as electrical interference can cause these devices to malfunction.
- Pacemaker devices must be checked prior to surgery and alternative pacing techniques (external or transvenous) and cardiac arrest trolley should be available.
- Surgical and theatre team must be informed.
- Bipolar is safer than monopolar diathermy.
- If monopolar diathermy is absolutely necessary, its use should be limited to short bursts. The neutral plate must be well adhered and sited as far away from the pacemaker as possible.
- ECG monitoring is paramount.

➤ **Monitor interference:**
- Diathermy interferes with monitoring including pulse oximetry, ECG and oesophageal Doppler.

What design features are incorporated within the diathermy system to minimise risk of electrical shock?

➤ **Use of an isolated patient circuit**
➤ **Use of an isolating capacitor:** Reactance of capacitors reduce with increasing current frequency. Therefore they have a higher impedance to low frequency currents (i.e. they block conduction of AC and minimise the risk of macro and micro shocks) but they have a lower impedance to high frequency diathermy currents (i.e. they allow conduction of these currents).

CHAPTER 59

Heat capacity and latent heat

Define freezing point

This is the temperature at which the liquid and solid phase of a substance of specified composition are in equilibrium at a given pressure.

Define boiling point

This is the temperature at which the liquid and vapour phase of a substance of specified composition are in equilibrium at a given pressure. When the vapour above the liquid is fully saturated the pressure it exerts (within a closed system) is called the saturated vapour pressure (SVP). When SVP equals the surrounding ambient pressure, the liquid begins to boil. Therefore, the boiling point is pressure dependent and this explains why you cannot make a nice hot cup of tea on top of Mount Everest (at sea level where the atmospheric pressure is 101.3 kPa water boils at 100°C but at the summit of Mount Everest where atmospheric pressure is 30 kPa water boils at about 80°C). In space water cannot be boiled as it just evaporates because the ambient pressure is zero (or very close to zero).

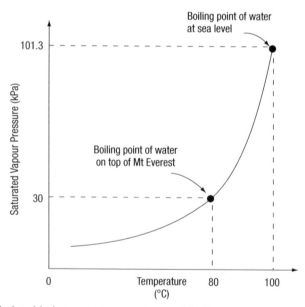

GRAPH 2.21 Relationship between temperature and SVP

Within a closed system, when the vapour pressure exceeds the ambient pressure, it pushes the vapour molecules back into the liquid and the liquid stops boiling. If the temperature increases further, the liquid boils and more molecules leave and the vapour pressure increases further. This increased vapour pressure pushes the molecules back into the liquid and the liquid stops boiling. This principle is utilised in the pressure cooker, which increases the boiling point of the substance by increasing the ambient pressure.

Draw a graph to depict the concept of latent heat and explain what happens

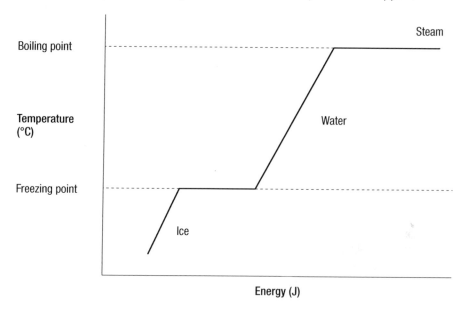

GRAPH 2.22 Temperature changes that occur when a block of ice changes phases as heat energy is applied

The graph above demonstrates the concept of latent heat:
➤ Latent heat refers to the amount of heat energy absorbed (or released) by a substance as it changes state at a specified temperature.
➤ As an object (e.g. block of ice) is given heat energy, its molecules will begin to vibrate more vigorously and the temperature of the object will increase (i.e. its kinetic energy increases).
➤ However, at the freezing and boiling points of the substance, any energy absorbed is not used to raise the object's temperature, but instead to increase the distance between its molecules (i.e. to increase its potential energy).
➤ Once the bonds are sufficiently weakened the molecules can move further apart and the substance can change phase.
➤ The amount of heat energy required to convert the phase of a substance from solid to liquid is known as the latent heat of fusion and from liquid into vapour is known as the latent heat of vaporisation.
➤ The specific latent heat of vaporisation (SLHV) is the energy required to change 1 kg of liquid into vapour.
➤ SLHV decreases with increasing temperature such that the SLHV of water at 37.5°C is 2.42 mJ/kg but at 100°C it is only 2.25 mJ/kg. However, there comes a point when no energy is required to change the state of a substance and this occurs at the critical temperature of that substance.

What clinical examples can you give where the concept of latent heat is important?
➤ Use of ethyl chloride to provide local anaesthetic – vaporisation of the agent causes cooling of the skin, rendering the area numb.
➤ Use of volatile anaesthetic agents – vaporisation of the agent leads to cooling which reduces the subsequent rate of vaporisation of the remaining agent and hence reduces

the SVP. Vaporisers therefore have temperature compensation mechanisms (e.g. bimetallic strip which adjusts the splitting ratio) incorporated into their design.

➤ Use of nitrous oxide cylinder and liquid oxygen contained with a vacuum-insulated evaporator – vaporisation of these agents leads to cooling which reduces the subsequent rate of vaporisation of the remaining agent and hence reduces the SVP.

➤ Loss of latent heat from the patient through warming and humidification of inspired gases.

➤ Loss of heat from the patient through evaporation.

What is the triple point of water?

It is the temperature (273.16 K or 0.01°C) and pressure (611.73 Pa or 0.006 atm) at which water exists in equilibrium in all three phases. It is a fixed point upon which the Kelvin scale of temperature is based.

What are the key concepts relating to SVP?

➤ The temperature at which SVP of a substance equals atmospheric pressure is the boiling point of that substance.

➤ For a given substance in a closed system, the SVP depends on temperature and nothing else.

➤ The maximum SVP of an open system at sea level is one atmosphere.

How can the SVP of water at altitude cause hypoxia?

If atmospheric pressure at altitude is 50 kPa and saturated water vapour pressure is 6.3 kPa, the above question can be answered using the alveolar gas equation:

$$P_{AMB}O_2 = F_{AMB}O_2 \times \textbf{Atmospheric pressure at altitude}$$
$$= 0.21 \times 50 \text{ kPa}$$
$$= 10.5 \text{ kPa}$$

$$PiO_2 = F_{AMB}O_2 \times \textbf{(Atmospheric pressure at altitude – SVP of water)}$$
$$= 0.21 \times (50 - 6.3)$$
$$= 9.17 \text{ kPa}$$

$$P_AO_2 = PiO_2 - P_ACO_2/RQ$$
$$= 9.17 - 5/0.8$$
$$= 2.92 \text{ kPa}$$

What are the effects of SVP on a vaporiser?

➤ As the vapour gets used up it is replaced by vaporisation of the volatile liquid.

➤ The process of vaporisation requires energy (latent heat of vaporisation).

➤ This energy requirement causes the temperature within the vaporiser to drop.

➤ As SVP is dependent on temperature, this causes the SVP of the vapour to also drop.

➤ In order to prevent this fluctuating SVP, vaporises have temperature-compensating mechanisms (e.g. bimetallic strip and wicks).

What are colligative properties?

Colligative properties are those properties of a solution that depend on the number of dissolved particles in a given mass of solvent and not on the identities and properties of those particles (i.e. they depend on the osmolality).

➤ **Freezing point** – 1 mole of solute added to 1 kg of water will reduce its freezing point by 1.86°C. This is why roads are gritted with salt during winter.

➤ **SVP** – solute particles occupy space within the solvent, reducing the surface area available for vaporisation and hence reducing SVP.

➤ **Boiling point** – this is the temperature at which liquid and vapour phases are in equilibrium but because solute particles occupy space within the solvent, the surface area available for solvent particles to enter the vapour phase is reduced. In order to re-establish equilibrium, the boiling point of the solution is achieved at a higher temperature. This is why salt added to a pan of pasta will hasten its cooking.

➤ **Osmotic pressure** – this is increased.

What is Raoult's law?

This law states that the depression of SVP of a solvent is proportional to the molar concentration of the solute present.

SVP

The easiest way to understand SVP is to imagine a saucepan half filled with a liquid on the hob. The lid is on the saucepan (i.e. it is a closed system) and the hob is switched off.

If left on the hob, some molecules of liquid inside the pan will escape the liquid phase, freeing themselves to become gaseous. Equally, some of the gaseous molecules will fall back into the liquid phase again. Once the system reaches equilibrium at a given temperature, (i.e. equal numbers of molecules leaving and entering the liquid/gas phase in a given time) the pressure inside this closed system is called the *SVP. Saturated* because the air in the container can hold no more gaseous molecules, *vapour* because the gas in the system is below its critical temperature and *pressure* because the 'banging' of the molecules against the side of the pan exerts a force per unit area.

If we now turn the hob on, we will deliver energy to the system. This will result in faster movement of its molecules. There will be more molecules escaping the liquid phase in a given time than before, though by definition, if in equilibrium, there will be more re-entering it. Because the molecules are moving faster with more energy, they will 'bang' against the sides of the container with more force, and so the pressure inside the system will be higher (think of the pan lid being lifted up by the bubbling water when you are cooking pasta on too high a heat.) This is why the SVP of liquid in a closed system will be greater at a higher temperature, and why we must always state the temperature when talking about SVP.

The SVP of a substance gives us an idea of how readily its molecules escape into the gaseous phase. If a substance evaporates or sublimates readily, it has a high SVP and is said to be 'volatile'.

Lastly, imagine a garden pond. This is an open system, as once the water molecules in the pond evaporate they can escape into the atmosphere. Hence, there is no container against which they can collide to create a pressure. The only pressure they must overcome to escape the liquid phase is the atmospheric pressure and so the SVP of an open system can only reach 1 atmosphere.

Pressure cookers utilise the concept of SVP. Here the lid is clamped on the container, and it will not allow the escape of air or liquid below a preset pressure. As defined above, the boiling point of a substance is when its SVP overcomes atmospheric pressure. Inside a pressure cooker, the atmospheric pressure is much higher than 1 and so the boiling point of water must be higher than 100°C. Consequently, food can be cooked more quickly because of the higher temperatures achieved. Conversely, you can't make a nice hot cup of tea on top Mt Everest because the low atmospheric pressure at that altitude means that water will boil at a temperature lower than 100°C.

CHAPTER 60

Temperature measurement

What is heat?
Heat is a form of energy associated with the kinetic motion of molecules within a substance. Heat energy gets transferred from a hotter to a colder substance.

What is temperature?
Temperature refers to the thermal state of a substance. It is the degree of 'hotness' of a substance and reflects its potential for heat transfer.

What is the SI unit of temperature?
The standard international unit of temperature measurement is the kelvin (K). It is based on the triple point of water, which is the temperature (at a specific pressure) at which water exists in all three phases (273.16 K or 0.01°C at a pressure of 611.73 Pa or 0.006 atm).
    1 unit kelvin = 1/273.16 of the thermodynamic triple point of water.
    A change in temperature of 1 K is equivalent to a change in temperature of 1°C.

	From Kelvin	To Kelvin
Celsius	[°C] = [K] –273.15	[K] = [°C] +273.15

(All calculations must be performed using the Kelvin scale and not Celsius. The volume of a gas will double only if the absolute temperature doubles. So if the temperature increases from 283.15 K (10°C) to 566.30 K (293.15°C) the gas volume will double but this will not apply if the temperature doubles from 10°C to 20°C!)

What methods can be used to measure temperature?
Temperature measurement can be divided into non-electrical, electrical and infrared-based methods.

Non-electrical:
➤ **Liquid expansion thermometers** (e.g. mercury and alcohol thermometers):
- **Principle:** Based on the volumetric expansion of a liquid with increasing temperature. Bulb containing the liquid is in communication with a narrow, linear, calibrated capillary tube. As the temperature increases the volume of the liquid expands and rises up the capillary tube. An angled constriction prevents the liquid contracting back into the bulb until shaken. Alternatively, a small bobbin sitting above the liquid gets left at the maximum reading point until the device is shaken.
- **Uses:** Mercury thermometers were previously used to measure body temperature (it freezes at about –39°C and boils at about 250°C) while alcohol thermometers are used to measure very low temperatures (alcohol freezes only at –114°C and boils at 78°C).
- **Advantages:** Cheap and easy to use.
- **Disadvantages:** Slow (2–3 min), glass thermometers can break causing injury and mercury is now classified as a hazardous substance.

➤ **Gas expansion thermometers** (e.g. Bourdon gauge dial thermometer):
  - **Principle:** Based on the volumetric expansion of a gas with temperature and the associated pressure changes that ensue due to this volume expansion. A bulb containing volatile liquid or saturated vapour is in communication with a hollow, elliptical, spiral tube. As the temperature rises, the volume in the bulb increases and as the hollow tube tries to accommodate the expanded gas it changes shape from elliptical to circular in order to give it the largest possible cross-sectional area. This shape change causes the tube to uncoil, moving a pointer across a temperature scale.
  - **Uses:** Used outdoors in harsh environments.
  - **Advantages:** Cheap, robust and gives continuous measurements.
  - **Disadvantages:** Poor accuracy and requires recalibration.
➤ **Bimetallic strip dial thermometer:**
  - **Principle:** Coil consisting of two different metals with different expansion coefficients. As the temperature increases these metals expand by different amounts, causing the coil to tighten, moving a pointer over the temperature scale.
  - **Uses:** Used outdoors in harsh environments.
  - **Advantages:** Cheap, robust and give continuous measurements.
  - **Disadvantages:** Poor accuracy and requires recalibration.
➤ **Chemical thermometer:**
  - **Principle:** Strip of small cells containing a chemical mixture that melts over a range of temperatures to produce temperature-dependent colour changes. Newer reusable models use liquid crystal technology, where tiny colourless, solid crystals melt with increases in temperature and then realign themselves, causing a colour change.
  - **Uses:** Clinical body temperature measurement.
  - **Advantages:** Fast response time (< 30s), disposable and no risk of glass breakage.
  - **Disadvantages:** Not extremely accurate at temperature differences less than 0.5°C.

Electrical:
➤ **Thermocouple:**
  - **Principle:** Consists of two different metals (e.g. copper and constantan, an alloy of copper and nickel) joined to form two separate junctions. One junction is kept at constant temperature and is known as the reference junction while the other junction acts as the temperature-measuring probe. When there is a temperature difference across these two junctions, a small voltage is produced. This voltage is proportional to the temperature difference across the junctions and is measured using a galvanometer. This phenomenon is known as the Seebeck effect.
  - **Advantages:** Rapid response time, accurate to within +/– 0.1°C and small.
  - **Disadvantages:** Voltage produced is very small and needs signal amplification and the reference junction needs to be at a constant temperature (or requires compensation).
➤ **Resistance thermometers** (e.g. platinum wire resistance thermometer):
  - **Principle:** Linear relationship between temperature and electrical resistance of a wire (e.g. platinum, copper or nickel) such that as temperature increases the resistance within a platinum wire increases in a predictable manner.
  - **Advantages:** Extremely accurate to within +/– 0.0001°C, with linear relationship between 0 and 100°C.
  - **Disadvantages:** Slow response time, bulky and fragile.

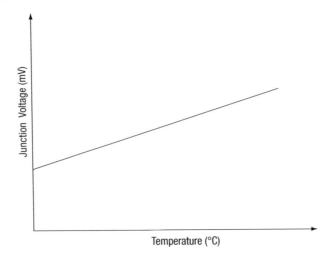

GRAPH 2.23 Change in junction voltage (mV) versus temperature (°C) for a thermocouple

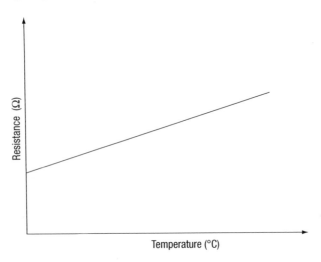

GRAPH 2.24 Change in resistance (ohms) versus temperature (°C) for a platinum resistance wire thermometer

➤ **Thermistor:**
  ● **Principle:** Semiconductor composed of heavy metal oxide (e.g. nickel, iron or manganese) which displays a negative exponential relationship between electrical resistance and temperature.
  ● **Uses:** Used clinically in PA catheters to measure core temperature.
  ● **Advantages:** Rapid response time (< 0.2 s), very small, accurate and cheap.
  ● **Disadvantages:** Hysteresis, ageing, variability within a batch and non-linear relationship requires recalibration.

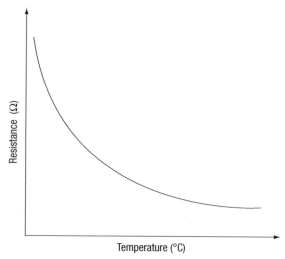

GRAPH 2.25 Change in resistance (ohms) versus temperature (°C) for a thermistor

Infrared:

➤ **Infrared tympanic membrane thermometers:**

- **Principle:** All living objects emit electromagnetic radiation, the wavelength of which is dependent on the temperature of that object. At body temperature, infrared radiation is the primary electromagnetic radiation given off by objects. Tympanic membrane thermometers receive infrared radiation from the tympanic membrane, which is close to the brain and therefore represents core body temperature. There are two main types of sensors that are used in these devices – the pyroelectric sensor and the thermopile sensor. The pyroelectric sensor contains crystals which alter their polarisation depending on the temperature. The thermopile sensor is made up of numerous thermocouples connected in parallel and allows continuous measurements to be made.
- **Uses:** Clinical measurement of core body temperature.
- **Advantages:** Non-invasive, accurate with a rapid response time ($< 5\,\text{s}$).

CHAPTER 61

Pollution and scavenging

Delivery of anaesthesia may result in atmospheric contamination by anaesthetic gases such as nitrous oxide and volatile agents. In 1996 the Health and Safety Executive agency placed constraints on the maximum allowable concentration of such substances within the theatre setting. In order to comply, scavenging of expired anaesthetic gases became mandatory.

What are the adverse effects of N_2O and volatile agents?
There are adverse effects to both the environment and to staff (and patients).
Environment:
➤ Volatile agents and N_2O are both known to damage the ozone layer.
➤ N_2O is also a 'greenhouse' gas contributing towards global warming.
➤ N_2O sustains combustion and therefore in the presence of lasers or grease it can become a fire hazard.

Staff (adverse effects are primarily related to the use of N_2O):
➤ **Bone marrow toxicity and peripheral neuropathy:** N_2O inhibits the enzyme methionine synthetase, which is involved in the synthesis of methionine (required for myelin formation) and tetrahydrofolate (required for DNA synthesis). It also oxidises the cobalt atom in vitamin B_{12} rendering it non-functional (vitamin B_{12} is a cofactor for methionine synthetase). The result is megaloblastic changes in bone marrow, bone marrow suppression, megaloblastic anaemia, impaired spinal cord myelination (subacute combined systems degeneration of the cord) and peripheral neuropathy.
➤ **Teratogenicity:** Exact mechanism is unclear but is likely to be multi-factorial and involve impaired DNA synthesis, which can manifest as neural tube defects.
➤ **Spontaneous miscarriage:** There were reports suggesting an increased incidence of miscarriages in dental practice nurses working with N_2O. Although these reports got a lot of publicity there is still no good level of evidence to support this observation.
➤ **Substance abuse**

What methods are available to reduce pollution in theatre?
➤ Air conditioning with rapid rate of air change (15 times per hour)
➤ Circle system
➤ Low gas flows
➤ Avoid using N_2O, use O_2 with air mix instead
➤ Scavenging systems
➤ Monitoring inspired and expired N_2O and volatile agent concentration and adjusting concentration to required clinical effect
➤ Monitoring theatre pollution levels
➤ Checking for leaks
➤ Capping breathing circuits when not in use (there is always a small leak)
➤ Vaporisers should be filled carefully to ensure no spillage
➤ Total intravenous anaesthesia technique

➤ Regional anaesthesia technique
➤ Rotate staff.

How can anaesthetic gases be scavenged?
Scavenging may be classified into active and passive systems.

Passive scavenging
➤ Requires no external power.
➤ Gas movement to the exterior is due to the pressure generated by the patient during expiration.
➤ This is an example of a ventile system (i.e. wind is used to entrain waste gases).

What are the problems with passive scavenging?
➤ Passive scavenging simply employs the use of wide-bore tubing to channel expired gases to the exterior and therefore it is not as effective as active methods.
➤ Excess positive or sub-atmospheric pressures may be caused by wind or air movement at the outlet.
➤ The outlets are above roof level to prevent re-entry of scavenged gas into the building. However, the weight of denser gases such as N_2O may exert a backpressure into the patient's breathing system.

Active scavenging
➤ Utilises an external power source such as vacuum pumps to generate a negative pressure, which propels gases to the external atmosphere.

What are the components of an active scavenging system?

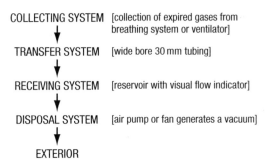

COLLECTING SYSTEM   [collection of expired gases from breathing system or ventilator]
↓
TRANSFER SYSTEM   [wide bore 30 mm tubing]
↓
RECEIVING SYSTEM   [reservoir with visual flow indicator]
↓
DISPOSAL SYSTEM   [air pump or fan generates a vacuum]
↓
EXTERIOR

➤ Gas from the expiratory valve of the breathing circuit or from the ventilator is collected and channelled via wide bore 30 mm diameter transfer tubing to the receiving system.
➤ The receiving system is usually an open-ended cylinder forming a reservoir for the collection of gases. The cylinder must be open ended as a safety precaution ensuring that the patient's airway cannot be subjected to excess positive or negative pressure.
➤ The receiving system also has a flow indicator. Scavenging flow rate is in the order of 80 L/min, which ensures removal of all expired gases.
➤ Gases in the reservoir are vented to the exterior atmosphere via a disposal system. The disposal system is either an air pump or fan. It operates within a pressures of −0.5 to + 5 cmH$_2$O.

What are the disadvantages of the active system?
➤ Excessive positive pressure may lead to barotrauma.
➤ Excessive negative pressure can deflate the reservoir bag of the breathing system and lead to rebreathing.

What is the recommended number of air changes per hour in theatre?

Despite scavenging, there will always be a quantity of gas that escape into the theatre environment, and therefore, the theatre needs adequate ventilation. Theatre ventilation should ensure 15 air changes per hour.

What is COSHH?

The Health and Safety Executive agency is a government agency with the role of preventing death, injury and ill health in Britain's workplaces. COSHH – Control of Substances Hazardous to Health sets safe maximum exposure limits to chemicals and other hazardous substances.

What are the maximum recommended anaesthetic pollutant levels?

These levels are based on an 8-hour TWA (time weighted average).

Halothane	10 ppm
Enflurane	50 ppm
Isoflurane	50 ppm
Nitrous oxide	100 ppm

No data is provided for sevoflurane or desflurane.

Are there any areas of the hospital in which long-term exposure limits may be difficult to achieve?

➤ It may be difficult to achieve acceptable pollution levels in post-anaesthesia care units – patients waking from anaesthesia with direct expiration into the environment of volatiles and possibly N_2O.

➤ Paediatric theatres – because of the use of non-closed breathing systems and high gas flows, e.g. Ayre's T-piece.

CHAPTER 62

Oxygen measurement

How may the concentration of oxygen in a gas mixture be measured?

There are multiple methods of measuring the concentration of oxygen in a gas mixture and it is essential to understand the principles behind each method. The different methods are:

➤ Clark polarographic electrode
➤ Galvanic fuel cell
➤ Paramagnetic O_2 analyser
➤ Mass spectrometer
➤ Photoacoustic spectroscope
➤ Raman spectroscope
➤ Chemical (e.g. Haldane apparatus).

Clark polarographic electrode:

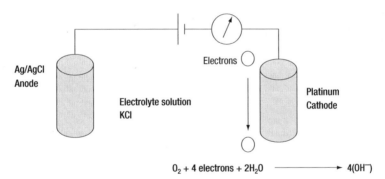

FIGURE 2.26 Schematic representation of Clark polarographic electrode

➤ Silver/silver chloride (Ag/AgCl) anode and platinum (Pt) cathode are suspended within a potassium chloride (KCl) solution.
➤ Voltage of 0.6 V is applied across the electrodes.
➤ Flow of current is measured.
➤ Anode reaction: electrons (e^-) are generated by the reaction of Ag^+ with the Cl^- ions from the KCl solution.
➤ Cathode reaction: O_2 combines with e^- and water to generate hydroxyl (OH^-) ions.

$$O_2 + 4e^- + 2H_2O \rightarrow 4(OH^-)$$

➤ The greater the amount of O_2 available, the greater the rate of electron uptake at the cathode and hence the greater the flow of current.
➤ Flow of current is therefore dependent on the O_2 tension at the cathode.
➤ Halothane may cause falsely high O_2 readings but this problem is overcome by the use of a halothane-impermeable membrane.

Galvanic fuel cell:

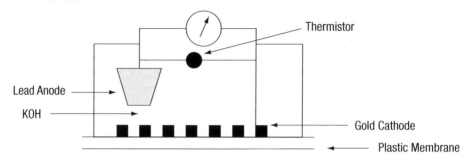

FIGURE 2.27 Schematic representation of galvanic fuel cell

➤ Similar in principle to the Clark polarographic electrode.
➤ Gold (Au) mesh cathode and lead (Pb) anode are suspended within a potassium hydroxide (KOH) solution.
➤ An electromotive force is produced.
➤ Anode reaction: electrons are generated from the reaction between OH^- from KOH and the Pb anode.

$$Pb + 2(OH^-) \rightarrow PbO + H_2O + 2e^-$$

➤ Cathode reaction: O_2 combines with electrons and water to generate hydroxyl ions (i.e. same reaction for the Clark electrode).

$$O_2 + 4e^- + 2H_2O \rightarrow 4(OH^-)$$

➤ Unlike the Clark electrode, no battery is required as the fuel cell generates its own voltage.
➤ Response time of the system is slow at approximately 30 s and therefore not suitable for breath to breath measurements.
➤ It has a limited lifespan of 6–12 months.
➤ Temperature compensation is achieved using a thermistor.
➤ Gas mixtures containing N_2O may damage the fuel cell. N_2O reacts at the lead anode, generating N_2, which alters the pressure within the cell potentially causing damage.

Paramagnetic oxygen analyser:
➤ O_2 is a paramagnetic gas, which means that it is attracted towards a magnetic field (due to unpaired electrons in its outer shell). Most other gases (e.g. N_2) are diamagnetic and are repelled from magnetic fields.
➤ Analyser is composed of two nitrogen-filled glass spheres connected in a dumbell arrangement, suspended from a filament within a gas-tight chamber. A mirror is attached to the dumbell.
➤ Glass spheres are subjected to a non-uniform magnetic field.
➤ If O_2 is added to the chamber, it is attracted towards the magnetic field, causing rotation of the glass spheres.
➤ The degree of rotation of the glass spheres can be measured using a simple light beam deflection principle. A beam of light passing to the mirror gets deflected as the mirror rotates. This deflected beam is sensed by a photodetector, which is calibrated to match the degree of rotation of the system to the oxygen concentration within the chamber.
➤ Newer versions use the null deflection principle. Instead of the glass spheres rotating, a current is supplied to oppose the movement of the spheres. The amount of current required to keep the spheres in their resting position is calibrated to O_2 concentration.

Mass spectrometer:

➤ Gas mixture is drawn into an ionising chamber where it is bombarded by electrons, which causes some of the gas molecules to become charged.
➤ Charged ions are then accelerated through a strong magnetic field which deflects these particles to varying degrees depending on their mass and momentum.
➤ Compounds of identical molecular weight (MW) are distinguished by identifying their breakdown products, e.g. N_2O and CO_2 both have MW 44 so N_2O is identified from its smaller nitric oxide fragment (MW 30).
➤ It has rapid response times of less than 0.1 s.
➤ It can measure a variety of gases within a mixture.
➤ Water vapour can interfere with the apparatus.
➤ It is a very bulky and an expensive piece of equipment.

Photoacoustic spectroscopy:

➤ Based on the photoacoustic effect, which was discovered by Alexander Graham Bell in his search for a means of wireless communication.
➤ Photoacoustic effect is the conversion between light and sound waves.
➤ Materials exposed to non-visible portions of the light spectrum (i.e. infrared and ultraviolet light) can produce acoustic waves.
➤ By measuring the sound at different wavelengths, a photoacoustic spectrum of a gas sample can be recorded which is used to identify the components within that sample.
➤ This effect can be used to study solids, liquids and gases.

Raman spectroscopy:

➤ When light interacts with a gas molecule the rotational and vibrational energy of the molecule is altered during the interaction. The resulting transfer of energy to or from the light changes its wavelength by amounts characteristic of the molecule concerned. Monochromatic radiation is therefore changed during its passage through a gas sample chamber into a spectrum of wavelengths, which depends on the structure of the individual gas molecules. Thus the type of molecules present and their concentrations in the gas sample can be determined.
➤ Raman effect is the scattering of a photon in a gas. Raman scattering can occur with a change in vibrational, rotational or electronic energy of a molecule.
➤ Raman spectroscope is composed of a helium–neon laser as its radiation source, a gas sample cell and a set of eight detectors, each with a specific radiation wavelength filter.
➤ Filters are manufactured to measure O_2, N_2, CO_2, N_2O and certain volatile agents.

Haldane apparatus:

➤ This is utilised as an instrument for estimating the proportion of oxygen in expired gases.
➤ It consists of a burette containing a volume of gas.
➤ The gas is then exposed to a solution of pyrogallol (a powerful reducing agent able to absorb oxygen).
➤ The volume of the remaining gas is then measured.
➤ The reduction in gas volume indicates the quantity of oxygen absorbed by the pyrogallol.
➤ This system can also be used to measure CO_2 but now a potassium hydroxide solution instead of pyrogallol is used.

pH measurement

Define pH
➤ pH stands for 'power of hydrogen'.
➤ It is a measure of the hydrogen ion activity in a solution.
➤ pH = negative log to the base 10 of hydrogen ion concentration [H$^+$], e.g. [H$^+$] of 10^{-7} mol/L = pH of 7.

There are a few rules of thumb worth remembering:
➤ Pure water is neutral and has a pH of 7.
➤ For each one unit change in pH there is a 10-fold change in [H$^+$].
➤ In the physiological range for each 0.3 change in pH there is a 50% change in [H$^+$].
    E.g. pH 6 = [H$^+$] 1000 nmol/L or 10^{-6} mol/L
        pH 7 = [H$^+$] 100 nmol/L or 10^{-7} mol/L
        pH 7.4 = [H$^+$] 40 nmol/L or $10^{-7.4}$ mol/L
        pH 8 = [H$^+$] 10 nmol/L or 10^{-8} mol/L
        pH 9 = [H$^+$] 1 nmol/L or 10^{-9} mol/L.

How is [H$^+$] measured?
Arterial blood gas analysers measure [H$^+$] and PCO_2 using potentiometric electrodes (i.e. voltage-producing electrodes) and PO_2 via an amperometric technique (i.e. current-producing electrodes).
    [H$^+$] is measured using a pH (glass) electrode, which is an ion-sensitive electrode whose operation depends upon the ion-sensitive glass at its tip.
    It is an example of a potentiometric electrode in that a potential difference develops across the ion-sensitive glass, the potential difference being dependent upon the difference in [H$^+$] across the glass.

Draw a simple schematic pH electrode
➤ Reference electrode: mercury/mercury chloride electrode within a potassium chloride solution. It indirectly makes contact with the blood sample via a membrane (permeable to only H$^+$).
➤ pH electrode: silver/silver chloride electrode within a buffer solution. The tip of the electrode is composed of ion-sensitive glass.
➤ System is maintained at 37°C as dissociation of acids and bases increases with increasing temperature.
➤ [H$^+$] is held constant around the pH electrodes by the buffer solution and hence any potential difference across this electrode are due to [H$^+$] within the blood sample.
➤ Electrical circuit must be completed between the blood sample and the two electrodes. In the case of the [H$^+$] ion electrode this is via the buffer and glass tip, while for the reference electrode this is via a membrane (avoids electrode contamination by the blood).

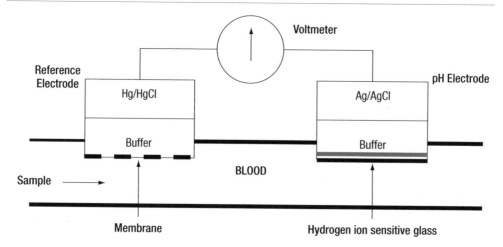

FIGURE 2.28 Schematic representation of pH electrode

➤ Potential difference between the two electrodes is measured and converted to a direct reading of pH or $[H^+]$.
➤ Potential output is linear (60 mV per unit pH).

How is the pH electrode calibrated?
The pH scale is not an absolute scale; it is relative to a set of standard solutions whose pH is established by international agreement. The system is calibrated using two buffer solutions, each containing a fixed concentration of phosphate buffers whose $[H^+]$ has been agreed by international agreement.

What are the sources of error in this measuring system?
The following conditions may result in erroneous $[H^+]$ results:
➤ Calibration errors
➤ Drift of the measuring system
➤ Membrane damage resulting in electrode contamination
➤ Temperature – hypothermia increases CO_2 solubility resulting in reduced $PaCO_2$ and increased pH
➤ Sampling errors
➤ Effect of over-heparinisation – acidic heparin lowers pH
➤ Delays in analysis of arterial blood gas – cellular metabolism continues:
  • PCO_2 rises about 0.009 kPa per minute
  • pH falls approximately 0.0006 units per minute
  • PO_2 falls approximately 0.13–0.39 kPa per minute

What other method can be used to measure pH?
A pH indicator is a substance that will change colour at a particular pH value (e.g. litmus paper turns red in acidic and blue in alkaline conditions).

CHAPTER 64

Carbon dioxide measurement

Carbon dioxide (CO_2) is routinely measured in anaesthetic practice:
➤ Arterial blood gas analysis (partial pressure of CO_2 in the blood)
➤ Capnography (percentage CO_2 in expired gas).

How is CO_2 measured in solution?
This is done using the Severinghaus CO_2 electrode.

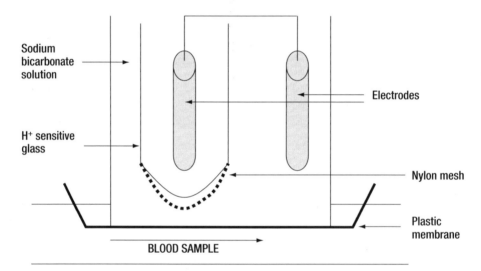

FIGURE 2.29 Schematic representation of Severinghaus CO_2 electrode

➤ Measurement of PCO_2 is based upon [H^+] measurement.

$$CO_2 + H_2O \leftrightarrow H_2CO_3 \leftrightarrow H^+ + HCO_3^-$$

➤ Severinghaus CO_2 electrode directly measures PCO_2 from the change in [H^+].
➤ Arterial blood sample is drawn into the system and remains separated from the nylon mesh via a plastic membrane.
➤ Plastic membrane is permeable to CO_2.
➤ CO_2 diffuses from the blood through the plastic membrane into the nylon mesh impregnated with the sodium bicarbonate solution.
➤ CO_2 combines with H_2O to generate H^+ ion and the resulting change in [H^+] is measured by the glass electrode (potentiometric electrode).
➤ Response time of the system is in the order of 2–3 min.
➤ Requires calibration prior to use with gas of known CO_2 concentration.

How is CO_2 measured in a gas mixture?

Capnography has become an integral part of monitoring in anaesthesia and helps to prevent life-threatening events. Monitors can use infrared spectrography, mass spectrography, Raman spectrography, photoacoustic analysers or colorimetric devices to measure carbon dioxide in the respiratory gases and then give a numerical reading (capnometry) and a waveform (capnography). We will look at the commonest monitor, the infrared analyser.

Infrared analyser
➤ Diatomic gas molecules (i.e. containing two or more different atoms) absorb infrared radiation.
➤ Each diatomic gas absorbs radiation of a particular wavelength.
➤ By measuring the proportion of infrared radiation absorbed by a gas mixture, the partial pressure of a diatomic gas can be measured.
➤ Infrared beam passes through a filter to obtain the required frequency for the gas of interest.
➤ Infrared beam splits and passes through reference and sample gas chambers.
➤ Sample and reference chamber windows are made of crystal (silver bromide or sapphire) as glass absorbs infrared.
➤ CO_2 absorbs infrared radiation and emergent beams are compared by photoelectric cells (the detector).
➤ Analyser is calibrated on air (assumed zero CO_2) and known concentration of CO_2 (gas cylinder) or electronically (step input voltage).
➤ Affected by barometric and extraction pressure in system – a change in atmospheric pressure directly influences the reading of capnographs since CO_2 concentration is measured as partial pressure.
➤ Water vapour trap required (water has high infrared absorbance).
➤ Hygroscopic tubing needed.

If you were allowed only one anaesthetic monitoring device what would you chose?

Most anaesthetists would probably request capnography because of the amount of information that can be gained from capnogram analysis:
➤ Confirmation of endotracheal intubation
➤ Detection of rebreathing (inadequate fresh gas flow)
➤ Detection of obstructive expiratory airflow
➤ Detection of inter-breathing in a ventilated patient
➤ Sudden fall in end-tidal CO_2 may indicate low systemic blood pressure, circulatory arrest or pulmonary embolism
➤ End-tidal CO_2 provides an estimation of arterial $PaCO_2$
➤ Detection of malignant hyperpyrexia

Which parameters are measured directly by an arterial blood gas analyser?

Directly measured:
➤ PaO_2
➤ $PaCO_2$
➤ pH

Derived:
➤ HCO_3^-
➤ Base excess
➤ O_2 saturations

CHAPTER 65

Blood pressure measurement

This is a common question both in the primary and final FRCA exam. Good basic understanding of the principles underlying BP measurement is essential.

How can you measure blood pressure?

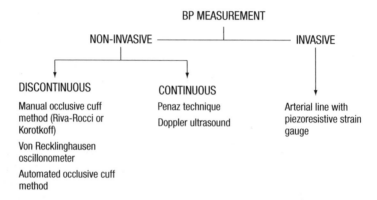

Describe the manual occlusive cuff method

This uses a cuff most commonly placed around the upper limb. The cuff must cover two-thirds of the length of the limb (or it must be 20% greater that the diameter of the limb). The width of a standard adult cuff is 14 cm and its length should be double its width. If the cuff is too small it will over-read and if too large it will under-read.

➤ **Riva-Rocci method:** Blood pressure was measured by palpation of the brachial or radial artery as the cuff was inflated. The loss of the pulse represented systolic blood pressure. Riva-Rocci (an Italian physician) was credited with developing the first conventional sphygmomanometer.

➤ **Korotkoff method:** Blood pressure was measured by auscultation over the brachial artery. In 1905, Korotkoff (a Russian army surgeon) described a series of noises that could be heard over the brachial artery as the cuff deflated:
  • **Phase I:** Tapping sound appears (systolic blood pressure)
  • **Phase II:** Sounds muffle or disappear (auscultatory gap)
  • **Phase III:** Sounds reappear with a tapping quality
  • **Phase IV:** Sounds muffle again (diastolic blood pressure in the UK)
  • **Phase V:** Sounds disappear (diastolic blood pressure in the USA). In a hyperdynamic circulation, the sounds may never disappear and this is why we use Phase IV to denote diastolic pressure.

What are the advantages and disadvantages of using this method?
Advantages:
➤ Simple
➤ No electricity required
➤ Doctor–patient contact

Disadvantages:
➤ Operator dependent
➤ Correct cuff size required
➤ Artefacts with arrhythmias and movement

How does a von Recklinghausen's oscillonometer work?
The old-fashioned versions of these machines work using two cuffs. The first is an occluding cuff, which sits proximally, and the second a sensing cuff against which the blood pulses once the occluding cuff has been deflated sufficiently to allow blood to flow under it. Each cuff is attached to two bellows and these bellow are attached to a single needle. A lever enables the operator to select which bellow's pressure is displayed by the needle (i.e. it can either make the needle 'sensing' or 'reading' depending on which position it is in).
➤ At systolic blood pressure – there is a sudden increase in needle oscillations.
➤ At mean arterial pressure – there is maximal amplitude in needle oscillations.
➤ At diastolic blood pressure – there is a sudden decrease in needle oscillations.

How does a 'DINAMAP' work?
DINAMAP® is the trade name for one of the original automated occlusive BP cuff measuring devices. It is based on the principle of an oscillonometer, but now the two cuffs have been merged into a single cuff, which performs both occluding and sensing functions. There is also a pneumatic pump, bleed valve, transducer, processor and display monitor.
➤ As the cuff deflates, the transducer detects the flow of blood under the cuff.
➤ The processor, with a built in algorithm, then relates the rate of change of pressure transients to systolic, diastolic and mean blood pressures.
➤ These readings are then displayed on the monitor.

Describe the Penaz technique (the 'Finapres')
Penaz principle states that 'the force exerted on a body can be determined by measuring an opposing force that prevents physical disruption'. It consists of an infrared plethysmograph within a pneumatic cuff.
➤ The Finapres cuff is wrapped around the distal phalanx of a finger (over a digital artery). It shines an infrared light through the finger, which is detected on the opposite side. The amount of light absorbed is directly proportional to the volume of the finger (this volume changes during systole and diastole).
➤ A pneumatic pump is controlled by the infrared signal. It continuously adjusts the cuff pressure in order to maintain a constant infrared signal (it aims to keep the volume of the finger constant, which represents the mean arterial pressure).
➤ The pressure inside the cuff required to achieve this is measured and gives a continuous arterial BP reading.

What are the advantages and disadvantages of this method?
Advantages:
➤ Continuous reading
➤ Accurate

Disadvantages:
➤ Downward drift due to tissue fluid relocation
➤ Painful after 20–30 min
➤ Ischaemia of digit

How can Doppler ultrasound be used to measure BP?
This is based on the principle of the Doppler shift.
➤ Transducer crystals within a probe transmit and receive ultrasound waves.
➤ Probe positioned over artery with a coupling medium (e.g. gel).
➤ As the arterial wall moves during systole and diastole there is a Doppler shift in frequency of the ultrasound waves (*see* question on 'Ultrasound').

What are the indications for direct arterial blood pressure measurement?
➤ When non-invasive BP measurements are inaccurate – obese, arrhythmias and during ambulance transfers.
➤ When extreme changes in blood pressure are expected – massive haemorrhage, cardiovascular instability and induced hypotension.
➤ When frequent arterial blood samples are required.
➤ When using pulse-contour cardiac output monitoring (e.g. LiDCO).

What are the components of an arterial line used to measure blood pressure?
➤ **Arterial cannula** – short, stiff and 20G size in adults
➤ **Tubing** – usually less than 120 cm, filled with 0.9% saline, connects cannula to transducer, must be free of kinks, clots and air bubbles
➤ **Three-way tap**
➤ **Pressurised fluid bag** – usually 0.9% saline, pressurised to 300 mmHg, with a drip rate of 4 mL/hr to prevent clot formation within the cannula
➤ **Piezoresistive strain gauge transducer** – must be zeroed to atmospheric pressure and kept at the level of the right atrium
➤ **Microprocessor, amplifier and display unit.**

What are the problems with invasive arterial blood pressure measurements?
➤ Cannula – disconnection leading to blood loss, infection, thrombosis and ischaemia (must check for collateral circulation, e.g. Allen's test).
➤ Transducer – calibration, resonance and damping.

Over-damping underestimates SBP, overestimates DBP but MAP remains the same (e.g. blood clot, air bubble or excessive tubing compliance). Under-damping overestimates SBP, underestimates DBP but MAP remains the same (e.g. tubing too long).

What other information can you obtain from an arterial waveform?
Heart rate, rhythm, MAP, stroke volume (area under curve), contractility (gradient of upstroke) and compliance of arterial tree (gradient of down stroke).

FORMULAE

$$MAP = \frac{SBP + (2 \times DBP)}{3}$$

$$DBP = \frac{(3 \times MAP) - SBP}{2}$$

CHAPTER 66

Cardiac output monitoring

Cardiac output (CO) is defined as the volume of blood ejected from the left ventricle per minute. It is determined by a number of interplaying factors including heart rate, rhythm, preload, contractility and afterload. Circulation (both in terms of pressure and flow) is essential to organ perfusion and O_2 delivery. However, it varies significantly under different physiological extremes and disease states.

Cardiac output monitoring measures various parameters associated with the central circulation and is currently the Holy Grail of haemodynamic assessment. Over the last decade there has been a rapid expansion in the use of CO monitoring devices within critical care and theatre settings to aid optimisation of haemodynamic variables and O_2 delivery and to facilitate goal-directed therapy.

The ideal method of measuring CO would be non-invasive, accurate, continuous, safe, easy to use and operator independent. It would provide rapid data acquisition and be cost-effective. Unfortunately, none of the currently available CO monitoring devices possesses all of these properties.

Conventional thermodilution techniques using a pulmonary artery floatation catheter (PAFC) remain the clinical gold standard for accuracy in CO monitoring. However, newer, less invasive monitoring devices that provide continuous cardiac output data are establishing a role in haemodynamic management.

What is the Fick principle?
➤ Fick (a nineteenth-century German physiologist, credited for Fick's law of diffusion and the invention of the contact lens) described the following relationship:

$$M = Q \times (A\text{-}V)$$

➤ The uptake or release of a substance (M) by an organ is the product of the blood flow (Q) through that organ and the arteriovenous concentration difference (A-V) of the substance in question.
➤ In essence, the Fick principle allows the blood flow to an organ (or the body) to be calculated using a suitable marker substance (e.g. dye, temperature or O_2).

How can you calculate CO using the Fick principle?
➤ The Fick method of calculating CO uses the Fick principle to measure the cardiac output of the pulmonary circulation.
➤ The A-V oxygen content difference across the lungs is measured via arterial and venous blood gases (i.e. a mixed venous sample from the pulmonary artery) and the rate of oxygen uptake is measured via spirometry.

$$\dot{V}O_2 = CO \times (CaO_2 - C\bar{v}O_2) \textbf{ and therefore } CO = \dot{V}O_2/(CaO_2 - C\bar{v}O_2)$$

Where:
$\dot{V}O_2$ = oxygen uptake
CaO_2 = arterial oxygen content

$C\overline{v}O_2$ = mixed venous oxygen content
CO = cardiac output

➤ In the absence of intra-pulmonary or intra-cardiac shunts, the pulmonary blood flow is equal to systemic blood flow and thus cardiac output.

What do you understand by the term 'assumed Fick determination'?
The Fick method is extremely accurate but in reality it is very time-consuming and cumbersome to obtain the required measurements. Therefore, the assumed value for O_2 consumption ($250\,mL/min$ or $125\,mL/min/m^2$) is sometimes used to calculate the CO. This is called an assumed Fick determination.

How is the dye or indicator dilution technique used to measure CO?
➤ A known quantity of dye (e.g. indocyanine green) or indicator substance (e.g. lithium) is injected into a central vein and then measured distally from a peripheral arterial blood sample.
➤ A graph of concentration over time is then plotted.
➤ However, due to recirculation of the substance, a second peak known as a recirculation hump is seen on the concentration time curves. This limits the total number of measurements that can be taken.
➤ The graph is therefore plotted semi-logarithmically in order to minimise the effect of this recirculation.
➤ The CO is inversely related to the area under this curve (AUC).
➤ Computer algorithms use the modified Stewart-Hamilton equation to calculate CO.

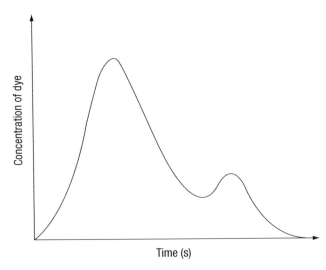

GRAPH 2.30 Concentration of dye over time

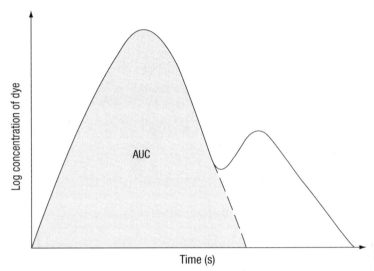

GRAPH 2.31 Log concentration of dye over time

What is a pulmonary artery flotation catheter (PAFC)?
➤ A PAFC is a device which can be used to measure cardiac filling pressures, pulmonary artery occlusion pressure, central venous oxygen saturations and core temperature.
➤ Cardiac output data may be acquired through thermodilution methods using the PAFC.
➤ Global use of the PAFC is falling as a result of newer, relatively less invasive methods of CO monitoring becoming available.
➤ Nevertheless, the PAFC is an extremely accurate method of CO monitoring and newer monitoring devices are routinely validated against the PAFC thermodilution technique.

Describe the key features of the PAFC
➤ Balloon-tipped, flow-directed catheter.
➤ 110 cm long.
➤ Inserted via a 5FG introducer sheath.
➤ Distal lumen should be positioned in the pulmonary artery (PA) to allow measurement of PA pressure and allow sampling of mixed venous blood.
➤ Proximal lumen is 30 cm from distal tip and should be positioned in the right atrium.
➤ Balloon at the tip is inflated with up to 1.5 mL of air (necessary to allow the catheter to advance with blood flow and to enable measurement of pulmonary capillary wedge pressure).
➤ Cardiac output is measured using cold thermodilution or pulsed heating bursts (latter available only in newer catheters).
➤ Pulmonary capillary wedge pressure (PCWP) provides an indication of left atrial filling pressure and thereby left ventricular end-diastolic pressure (LVEDP) which is used as a surrogate for left ventricular end-diastolic volume (LVEDV) which represents preload.

How is cardiac output measured using a PAFC?
➤ A thermodilution technique is used (which is an advance on the dye dilution technique) where heated or cooled fluid is now used to replace the dye.

➤ This eliminates the problems of recirculation, allowing infinite measurements to be made.

➤ 10 mL of ice-cold 0.9% saline (or 5% dextrose) is injected via the proximal port of the PAFC into the right atrium, thereby reducing the blood temperature.

➤ The blood temperature is then measured by a distal thermistor on the PAFC and a thermodilution curve (temperature change against time) is generated.

➤ Cardiac output is inversely related to the AUC and computer programmes calculate it using the **Stewart-Hamilton equation**:

$$Q = \frac{V\ (T_B - T_I)\ K_1\ K_2}{T_B\ (t)\ dt}$$

Where:

Q	cardiac output
V	volume of injectate
T_B	temperature of blood
T_I	injectate temperature
$K_1 K_2$	computer constants
$T_B\ (t)\ dt$	change in blood temperature over time

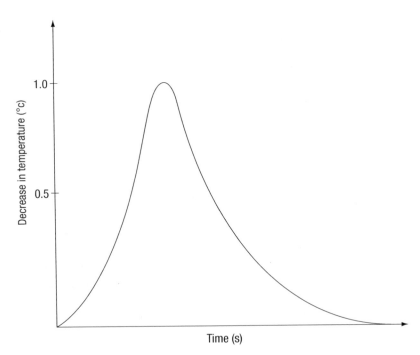

GRAPH 2.32 Change in temperature over time

➤ Modern PAFCs are able to provide continuous CO data. They contain an electric heating coil which is positioned in the right atrium and which heats up the blood in a semi-random fashion. The pulsed heating bursts are detected by the thermistor and via the same Stewart-Hamilton method CO is calculated.

Draw a pressure trace to illustrate the PAFC passage to the pulmonary artery

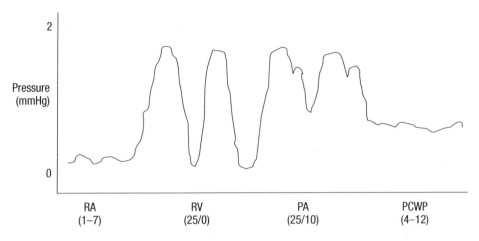

FIGURE 2.33 PAFC passage through the heart

In what circumstances does PCWP overestimate LVEDP?
Any condition creating an interfering pressure gradient which does not represent function of the left ventricle:
➤ Mitral stenosis
➤ Positive end expiratory pressure (PEEP)
➤ Pulmonary hypertension.

In what circumstances does PCWP underestimate LVEDP?
Any condition causing increased pressure within the left ventricle, which the catheter tip cannot detect:
➤ Poorly compliant left ventricle
➤ LVEDP > 25 mmHg.

How is a PCWP of 25 mmHg interpreted?
➤ The most common interpretation of an elevated PCWP in the assumed setting of normal juxtacardiac pressure and normal ventricular compliance would be that of hypervolaemia with an increased LVEDV causing an elevated PCWP.
➤ However, if juxtacardiac pressure is increased as in cardiac tamponade or constrictive pericarditis, the same elevated PCWP may be associated with normal or reduced LVEDV.
➤ Another scenario is possible if ventricular compliance is reduced (e.g. diastolic dysfunction arising from myocardial ischaemia), in which case again LVEDV may be normal or reduced despite elevated PCWP.
➤ These problems delineate the basis of arguments that are now made against the use of PCWP as a marker of fluid responsiveness.

What other methods of cardiac output measurement do you know of?
Examiners will expect an understanding of the principles behind cardiac output monitoring and may wish to explore the advantages and disadvantages of some of the commoner technologies available.

Non-invasive techniques:

➤ **Transcutaneous Doppler** (e.g. ultrasound cardiac output monitor – USCOM)
  - Based on the Doppler effect.
  - Transcutaneous probe is placed on the supra-sternal notch of the patient.
  - Measures blood flow in the pulmonary artery and across the semi-lunar valves.
  - Device plots velocity of trans-valvular and trans-pulmonary blood flow over time.
  - Programmed algorithms within the device then calculate the CO.
  - User-dependent and requires training.
➤ **Transthoracic electrical bioimpedance**
  - Based on the principle that during ejection of blood from the heart in systole there is an associated change in electrical impedance of the thoracic cavity due to the increased blood volume, the rate of change of this impedance is a reflection of CO.
  - Four dual electrodes or sensors are placed on the neck and thorax and a low current is passed between them.
  - Current seeks the path of least resistance, which in this case is the blood-filled aorta.
  - Blood volume and velocity within the aorta changes from beat to beat and this equates to changes in thoracic impedance.
  - Device measures the corresponding changes in impedance and relates this to CO.
  - Quick to set up and easy to use.
  - Useful in estimating trends in CO but not for absolute measurements.
  - Studies suggest the method is accurate in healthy volunteers, but its reliability decreases in critically ill patients.
  - Technique has not gained wide clinical acceptance.
➤ **Non-invasive cardiac output monitor (NICO)**
  - Applies the Fick principle to CO_2.
  - Changes in CO_2 concentration after intermittent periods of partial rebreathing through a special rebreathing loop are measured.
  - Sensors are placed to measure CO_2, air flow and airway pressures.
  - $\dot{V}CO_2$ is calculated from minute ventilation including its CO_2 content while $PaCO_2$ is estimated from end tidal CO_2 measurements.
  - System relies solely on airway gas measurement.
  - Calculates effective lung perfusion (i.e. that part of the pulmonary capillary blood flow that has passed through ventilated parts of the lung).
  - Effects of unrecognised ventilation–perfusion inequality in patients may explain why the results with this method show a lack of agreement with thermodilution techniques.

Invasive techniques:

➤ **Transoesophageal Doppler**
  - Based on the Doppler effect.
  - Velocity of blood flow in the descending thoracic aorta is measured using a flexible ultrasound probe placed in the mid-oesophagus.
  - Nomograms are used to calculate diameter of the descending aorta (based on height, age and weight).
  - Provides indicator of preload (flow time corrected to 60 beats per min) and contractility (peak velocity and mean acceleration).
  - Systemic vascular resistance is calculated.
  - Rapid data acquisition.

- Only measures blood flow in the descending aorta and hence flow to head, neck and upper limbs is excluded.
- Not tolerated by awake patients.
- Suffers interference from surgical diathermy.
- Operator dependent and requires skill to align probe and obtain good signal.
- Contraindicated in those with oesophageal varices.
- Risk of oesophageal perforation.

➤ **Dye and temperature dilution techniques** (covered previously)
- Based on the Fick principle.
- Injection of a substance into the right side of the heart and detection of the same substance distally, either in the pulmonary artery or in the systemic circulation.
- Concentration-time (or temperature–time) curve is generated.
- CO is calculated via the Stewart-Hamilton equation and AUC.

➤ **Arterial pulse pressure contour analysis** (e.g. PiCCO and LiDCO)
- Based on arterial pulse contour analysis, it uses the arterial waveform and pressures to calculate stroke volume and CO.
- Fluctuations of blood pressure around its mean value occur as a specific volume of blood, the stroke volume (SV), is ejected into the aorta by each contraction. The magnitude of this pressure change, the pulse pressure, is a function of the magnitude of the SV. Thus on a beat-to-beat basis, the only factor that determines changes in pulse pressure is a change in SV.
- Requires insertion of an arterial line (special femoral arterial line required for PiCCO).
- Not reliable with arrhythmias.
- Physiological and therapeutic changes in vessel wall diameter are assumed to reflect changes in cardiac performance – this effect is minimised by intermittent calibration.
- PiCCO device is calibrated via a transpulmonary thermodilution technique.
- LiDCO device is calibrated via a lithium dilution technique.
- PiCCO device identifies the systolic area by recognising the dicrotic notch on the arterial waveform. Systolic area is by definition the stroke volume. It is converted to an absolute number by calibration.
- In addition to CO and SV, PiCCO device also provides 'dynamic' indicators of volume responsiveness: stroke volume variation (SVV), pulse pressure variation (PPV), systolic pressure variation (SPV) as well as a number of volumetric markers of preload: global end-diastolic volume, intrathoracic blood volume and extravascular lung water.
- LiDCO utilises an existing arterial line and tracks the power of the arterial waveform rather than the contour in order to track changes in SV.
- Theoretical advantage of LiDCO is the reduction of the effect of reflected waves because the device does not need to identify specific parts of the arterial waveform.
- LiDCO calibration is not possible in the presence of atracurium.
- LiDCO also provides dynamic indicators of preload (SVV, SPV and PPV).

CHAPTER 67

Depth of anaesthesia monitoring

The definitions and management of awareness are dealt with in *Study Guide 2*, Part 3, 'Critical Incidents', Chapter 47, 'Awareness'.

How can the depth of anaesthesia be monitored?

To date there is no agreed 'gold' standard against which techniques or equipment used to monitor depth of anaesthesia can be tested. Over the years, there have been many methods proposed for monitoring depth of anaesthesia, but few are used with any regularity. Currently, there is no single method that can consistently and reliably monitor depth of anaesthesia.

➤ **Clinical methods:**
  - **Clinical signs** – in the spontaneously ventilating patient, movement and the depth and frequency of respiration are useful indicators of anaesthetic adequacy. In the paralysed patient these features are lost and instead signs of sympathetic stimulation are often used. The PRST (or Evan's) scoring system (pressure, rate, sweating and tears) was developed to provide an objective assessment of sympathetic stimulation. However, the scoring system is not specific to the effects of anaesthesia and absence of sympathetic activity does not exclude awareness.

➤ **Instrumental methods:**
  - **Tunstall's isolated forearm technique** – a tourniquet is applied to the arm prior to induction of anaesthesia with the assumption that any muscle relaxant will therefore not reach the muscles of the arm. If the patient is aware, they will be able to move their hand to alert the anaesthetist. This is mainly a research tool and studies have shown a poor correlation with recall after the event.
  - **Lower oesophageal contractility** – a balloon catheter with a distal pressure transducer is placed in the lower oesophagus. Provoked oesophageal contractions are triggered by inflation of the balloon while spontaneous oesophageal contractions are triggered by stress and emotion in an awake patient. These contractions are recorded by the pressure transducer and using an algorithm the device generates the oesophageal contractility index for that patient.
  - **Bispectral index (BIS) monitor** – this is currently the most commonly used technique. An electrode strip is placed on the patient's forehead and cortical activity is recorded in the form of an electroencephalogram (EEG). This data is analysed by the BIS machine to produce a dimensionless number, which is supposed to correlate with depth of anaesthesia. When the patient is awake, cerebrocortical activity is increased with more higher frequency signals generated. This leads to the generation of a higher number:

    100–85 Awake and capable of explicit recall
    85–60   Increasing sedation, impaired memory processing but rousable with stimulation

60–40   Surgical anaesthesia where auditory processing and reflex movement are still possible but memory is less likely

40–0   Burst suppression (0 = electrical silence)

The BIS algorithm was found by analysing the EEG in healthy volunteers who were in various degrees of consciousness from awake, through to sedated and anaesthetised. The trial was repeated on a second cohort of healthy subjects, and then on patients. Blinded studies have shown that most anaesthetists will give a general anaesthetic with a BIS of 30–40 when using the monitor.

- **Power Spectral Analysis (PSA)** – this is also based on EEG analysis. The raw EEG data undergoes Fourier's analysis to break it down into its constituent sine waves. These are then processed and displayed graphically. The 'power' wave amplitude drops as the depth of anaesthesia increases. There are problems with inter-patient variability.
- **Auditory Evoked Potentials (AEP)** – this has evolved on the basis that the auditory sense disappears last when undergoing anaesthesia. A series of clicks is delivered into the patient's ear as they are anaesthetised. The resulting EEG is monitored and analysed to give an AEP index (AEP > 80 is awake and AEP < 50 is asleep). Unlike BIS monitoring, the system exhibits much less hysteresis and there are defined 'awake' and 'asleep' points. It is now being marketed with an algorithm giving arbitrary values of 0–100.
- **Raw EEG** – this can be accurate but needs expert interpretation.

How reliable is BIS monitoring?

There are several problems with trusting the BIS algorithm:

➤ The patients used in the trials to produce the algorithm were anaesthetised using only hypnotics. The effect of adding opiates to the induction was not studied.

➤ Most of the studies did not include giving the patients a surgical stimulus, therefore the BIS number cannot be said to correlate accurately with surgical anaesthesia.

➤ The studies were only performed on adults and so the data cannot confidently be extrapolated to children < 5 years old.

➤ There is variability between patients, and a BIS number that may render one patient 'asleep' to a surgical stimulus may allow movement in another.

➤ It is not possible to predict from the BIS number at what point the patient will be anaesthetised, nor when they will wake up.

In what other settings might a BIS monitor be used?

BIS can be used on the intensive care unit to monitor burst suppression, which is a technique used to reduce cerebral metabolic oxygen requirements in patients with head injuries, raised intracranial pressures or in status epilepticus.

BIS can also be used on the intensive care unit to reduce awareness in those paralysed for long periods of time.

CHAPTER 68

Safety features of the anaesthetic machine

Despite the advances in technology and the development of newer and more sophisticated anaesthetic machines, it is still an essential requirement to understand the safety features governing the use of such devices.

What are the principal functions of the anaesthetic machine?
➤ Accurately and continuously deliver a gas and volatile mixture of the desired composition
➤ Avoid delivering hypoxic gas mixtures
➤ Avoid causing barotrauma to the patient.

What are the safety features of an anaesthetic machine?
In order not to miss anything, it is best to start from the wall where the pipeline supply commences and then work systematically from the back of the machine to the common gas outlet.
➤ All anaesthetic machines should be checked prior to use by the anaesthetist.
➤ Colour coded gas pipes (black = air, white = oxygen and blue = nitrous oxide) connect to the wall via a Schraeder valve (gas specific and non-interchangeable) and connect to the back of the anaesthetic machine via non-interchangeable screw threads (NIST – gas specific and permanently fixed).
➤ Colour coded gas cylinders (oxygen = black body with white shoulder, nitrous oxide = blue body with blue shoulder and air = black body with white and black shoulders) act as an emergency source of gases should primary piped gas delivery fail. They connect to the back of the anaesthetic machine via a pin-indexed system (oxygen = 2.5, nitrous oxide = 3.5 and air = 1.5) incorporating a Bodok seal to make the connection gas-tight.
➤ Pressure regulators reduce the pressure of cylinder gases to approximately 400 kPa (i.e. the same as piped gas pressure), thereby protecting the anaesthetic machine from damage due to high gas pressures.
➤ Flow control needle valves allow fresh gas flow to be regulated. The control knobs are labelled and colour coded. The oxygen control knob is larger, protrudes further and is grooved to allow differentiation from the air and nitrous oxide control knobs. An anti-hypoxic link prevents delivery of a hypoxic gas mixture by linking the nitrous oxide flow to a minimum oxygen flow.
➤ Rotameters are constant pressure, variable orifice flowmeters, which allow fresh gas flow rates to be measured (calibrated to individual gases as the density and viscosity of the gases are important). Oxygen is the last gas to be added to the fresh gas flow, which prevents delivery of a hypoxic gas mixture should a proximal crack in the flowmeter occur. Rotamaters are produced with anti-static material to prevent the bobbin 'sticking', which could result in inaccurate fresh gas flow measurement.
➤ Back-bar pressure relief valves are situated downstream of the vaporisers and vent off

gas mixtures at pressures greater than 35 kPa. This prevents barotrauma to the flow meters and vaporisers but not the patient.

➤ Oxygen supply failure alarm is activated when the oxygen supply pressure falls below 2 bar. It produces a sound of at least 60 dB for a minimum 7 seconds. Activation relies solely on oxygen pressure and when oxygen supply failure has occurred, flow of all other gases cease and atmospheric air is entrained.

➤ Oxygen flush provides 100% oxygen at flow rates between 40–75 L/min and at a pressure of about 400 kPa. This bypasses the flowmeters and vaporisers.

➤ Vaporisers convert volatile liquid into vapour and add a controlled amount of volatile to the fresh gas flow. Selectatec vaporiser interlocking mechanisms prevent the use of more than one vaporiser at any one time, thereby avoiding contamination of a downstream vaporiser. Vaporiser filling devices are geometrically coded and agent specific, designed to prevent incorrect vaporiser filling.

➤ Vital monitoring adjuncts include oxygen concentration analysers, inhalational agent concentration analysers, end-tidal carbon dioxide analysers, high airway pressure alarms and ventilator disconnection alarms.

CHAPTER 69

Breathing systems

A question on breathing systems often starts with the examiner showing photographs of different types of system, asking you to identify them and explain how they function.

There are three main objectives when using a breathing system:

➤ To supply O_2 to the patient
➤ To allow removal of CO_2 from the system and avoid rebreathing
➤ To supply anaesthetic gases to the patient.

There are several classification systems, but the most commonly used (and examined) is the Mapleson classification system (Professor Bill Mapleson worked in Cardiff and classified the breathing systems in 1954).

Describe the movement of gas within each system

The respiratory cycle comprises three phases: inspiration, expiration and the expiratory pause.

➤ During inspiration, gas is drawn in from the equipment.
➤ In quiet breathing, the average 70 kg patient's tidal volume is approximately 500 mL. At 20 breaths per minute, their minute volume (MV) would be 10 L/min. In order to avoid rebreathing, the fresh gas flow rate would have to exceed the patient's MV. This would result in very high volumes of gas needing to be delivered. This is wasteful and requires high flow rates that would be uncomfortable for the patient.
➤ With maximum effort, the average 70 kg patient can draw in approximately 5 L of gas over about 2 seconds. Again, unless flow rates were extremely high the patient would entrain air.
➤ To overcome these problems, reservoir bags have been added to the breathing systems.
➤ During deep inspiration the patient can draw oxygen and gases from these as well as from the fresh gas flow.
➤ At the beginning of expiration, gas expired is from the anatomical dead space, so it does not contain CO_2 and is not depleted of O_2. This gas is fit to be inhaled again.
➤ As expiration continues, alveolar gas is exhaled next, this contains CO_2 and is O_2 deplete. It is desirable to rid the system of this gas before the next inspiration.
➤ Adjustable pressure-relieving (APL) valves have been added to some circuits to vent waste gases and overcome the problem of rebreathing.

MAPLESON A (Non-co-axial 'Magill' system)
Spontaneous ventilation

When describing breathing systems always start with the statement, 'The patient has just exhaled, the equipment is full of fresh gas and I put the mask over the patient's face. At the perfect flow rate . . .'

➤ The patient inhales fresh gas, from the supply and from the reservoir bag, which deflates proportionally.
➤ The patient exhales and the dead space volume is expelled into the breathing system,

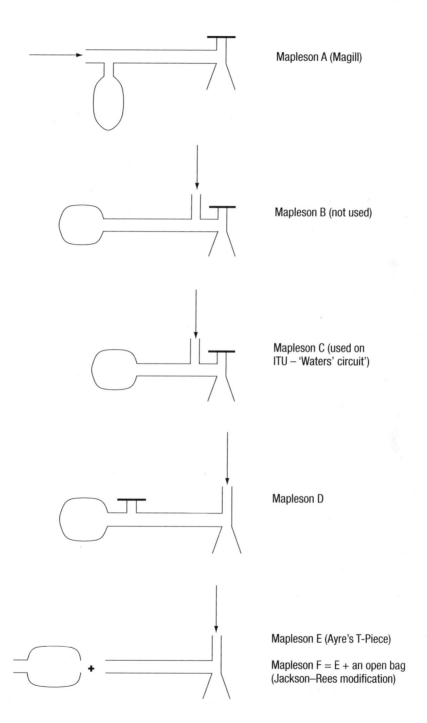

Mapleson A (Magill)

Mapleson B (not used)

Mapleson C (used on
ITU – 'Waters' circuit')

Mapleson D

Mapleson E (Ayre's T-Piece)

Mapleson F = E + an open bag
(Jackson–Rees modification)

FIGURE 2.34 Diagrammatic representation of Mapleson classification of breathing systems
(the arrow represents the entry of fresh gas)

passing down the tubing and fills the reservoir bag again. In addition the fresh gas flow will also contribute to filling the bag.

➤ After the dead space gas, the alveolar gas is exhaled. At this stage the reservoir bag is already filled and so the pressure in the system begins to rise. Because of this, the alveolar gas is vented through the APL valve and lost from the system, so avoiding rebreathing.

➤ If the fresh gas flow is too low, the bag will not be filled solely by dead space gas. Some alveolar gas will be able to enter the bag, and the patient will rebreathe.

➤ If the fresh gas flow is too high, the fresh gas flow will fill the bag to a degree and dead space gas will be vented along with alveolar gas. While this avoids rebreathing, it is wasteful and inefficient.

Controlled ventilation

➤ The anaesthetist squeezes the bag, forcing gas into the patient. Some gas, however, will be vented from the expiratory valve near the patient. At the end of inspiration, the reservoir bag will not be full.

➤ During exhalation, dead space and alveolar gas will move down to fill the reservoir bag.

Unless the gas flows are high, 2.5 × MV, rebreathing will occur.

The Mapleson A is:

➤ Efficient in spontaneous ventilation (70 mL/kg/min)

➤ Inefficient for controlled ventilation (2.5 × MV).

MAPLESON A (Co-axial version 'Lack' system)

Co-axial means there is an inner tube surrounded by an outer one.

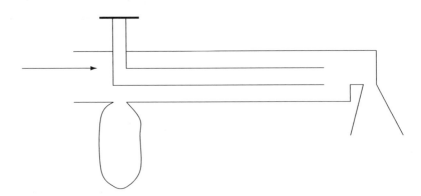

FIGURE 2.35 Co-axial Mapleson A

The Lack is a version of the Mapleson A, which was designed to move the pressure release valve away from the patient and so make it less awkward and bulky to use. The fresh gas flows down the outside tubing, and gas is vented via the inner tubing. The reservoir bag is in the inspiratory limb, while the pressure release valve is in the expiratory limb. The gas flows required in the system are the same as for the standard A. The Lack is bulkier than the Bain (*see* next page) because the inner tube has to have a sufficiently large diameter to minimise expiratory resistance.

MAPLESON B and C

These are essentially the same, but the C has shorter tubing. The B is not used. The C is used for transfer, or 'bagging' patients on ICU. This system needs high gas flows to prevent rebreathing (2.5 × MV for spontaneous and controlled ventilation).

The Mapleson C is colloquially referred to as a 'Waters' circuit', though strictly this is inaccurate as a true Waters' circuit would include a canister of soda lime to absorb CO_2 and prevent rebreathing. These are not manufactured any more.

MAPLESON D (Non-co-axial system)

Spontaneous ventilation

The patient has just exhaled, the equipment is full of fresh gas and I put the mask over the patient's face. At the perfect flow rate . . .

➤ The patient inhales fresh gas, from the supply and from the reservoir bag, which deflates proportionally.

➤ The patient exhales and the dead space volume is expelled into the breathing system. The fresh gas flow and the exhaled dead space gas mix and both pass down the tubing to fill the reservoir bag.

➤ After the dead space gas, the alveolar gas is exhaled. At this stage the reservoir bag is already filled and so the pressure in the system begins to rise. Because of this, the alveolar gas is vented through the pressure release valve and lost from the system so avoiding rebreathing.

➤ During the expiratory pause, fresh gas continues to push exhaled alveolar gas down towards the reservoir bag (as the pressure release valve is further away than in the A) and rebreathing will occur at gas flows of < 2.5 × MV.

Controlled ventilation

➤ The patient exhales and a mixture of fresh gas and dead space gas enter the bag, as described above.

➤ The anaesthetist squeezes the bag and fresh gas from the distal tubing is forced into the patient and a variable amount of gas from the reservoir enters the patient. Following this, the pressure in the system rises (according to the patient's lung compliance) and further gas gets vented from the expiratory valve.

The Mapleson D is:

➤ Inefficient for spontaneous ventilation (2.5 × MV)

➤ Efficient for controlled ventilation (70 mL/kg/min)

MAPLESON D (Co-axial 'Bain' system)

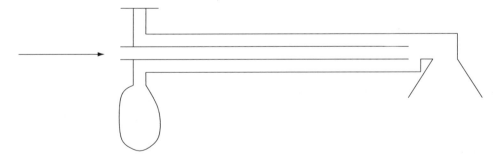

FIGURE 2.36 Co-axial Mapleson D

In this circuit the fresh gas flows down the inner tubing, and exhaled gas enters the outer tubing. Both the reservoir bag and APL valve are in the expiratory limb. The Bain is equally efficient for controlled or spontaneous ventilation.

During controlled ventilation at a flow rate of 70 mL/kg/min, the patient will in fact be rebreathing. However, because we tend to over-ventilate our patients, their end tidal CO_2 will not actually rise despite the fact they are rebreathing. If we managed not to over-ventilate, we would actually see a rising E_TCO_2 as evidence of this. To truly avoid rebreathing during controlled ventilation in the Bain circuit we would need to use 2.5 × MV, the same flow rate as is necessary to avoid it in spontaneous ventilation.

MAPLESON E
This is also called the Ayre's T-Piece after the man who invented it.

It has no valves or reservoir bag and so is a very low resistance system. This makes it suitable for use in paediatrics.

MAPLESON F
This is an E with the 'Jackson-Rees modification' – an open-ended reservoir bag connected to the end of the tubing. This allows for the application of CPAP and controlled ventilation.

In both E and F, fresh gas flows of 2.5 × MV are required to prevent rebreathing.

TABLE 2.37 Volume of fresh gas flow required to prevent rebreathing during spontaneous and controlled ventilation using the Mapleson breathing systems.

Mapleson classification	Spontaneous ventilation	Controlled ventilation
A	70 mL/kg/min	2.5 × MV
B	2.5 × MV	2.5 × MV
C	2.5 × MV	2.5 × MV
D	2.5 × MV	70 mL/kg/min
E	2.5 × MV	2.5 × MV
< 20 kg	2.5 × MV (minimum 3 L/min)	1000 mL + 100 mL/kg/min

CHAPTER 70

Resuscitation bags and valves

Questions about the above will revolve around non-rebreathing valves so it is essential to be able to name, describe and even draw the various types.

What type of resuscitation bag do you find on a cardiac arrest trolley?
A self-inflating bag with a non-rebreathing valve and mask is found on a cardiac arrest trolley. This is a compact and portable ventilating system that does not require a pressurised gas supply to work. It consists of a fresh gas inlet with a one-way valve (commonly in communication with an O_2 reservoir bag to increase FiO_2), an entrainment valve at the inlet (to allow entrainment of air if oxygen supply does not meet respiratory demands), a self-inflating bag (1500 mL for adults, 500 mL for children and 250 mL for infants), a non-rebreathing valve and a pressure relieving valve to prevent barotrauma.

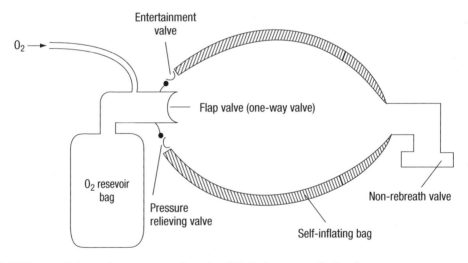

FIGURE 2.38 Schematic representation of self-inflating resuscitation bag

How does it work?
The main component in a self-inflating resuscitation bag is the non-rebreathing valve (e.g. Reuben, Ambu E and Laerdel valves). Their function is to ensure that gas flows out of the self-inflating bag and into the patient during inspiration and that exhaled patient gases pass out through the expiratory port and do not re-enter the self-inflating bag.

Non-rebreathing valves are made up of the following:
➤ Inspiratory port, often coloured blue ('blue to bag'), supplying fresh gas for inspiration.
➤ Expiratory port, often coloured yellow or gold ('gold for go'), allowing the exit of exhaled gases.
➤ Patient port that connects to the airway adjunct (mask, LMA, OETT).
➤ One-way valve or valves ensuring exhaled gases are not rebreathed.

Reuben valve:

➤ This consists of a spring-loaded bobbin.

➤ During positive pressure ventilation, as the bag is squeezed, the bobbin is pushed across and closes the expiratory port, allowing fresh gas to enter the patient.

➤ During expiration, as the bag relaxes, the bobbin shifts to the opposite side and closes the inspiratory port, allowing exhaled gases to escape through the expiratory port.

➤ The bag then self-inflates, drawing in air from the room and oxygen from the reservoir bag ready to deliver the next breath.

➤ The valve can jam, keeping the inspiratory port continuously open, which risks hyperinflating the lungs.

➤ The valves offer resistance ($0.8\,cmH_2O$ during inspiration and $1\,cmH_2O$ during expiration) and therefore can significantly increase the work of breathing and impair passive expiration in the spontaneously ventilating patient. Therefore, these devices should be used cautiously in patients with respiratory fatigue ('assisted' breaths should be given to such patients by gently squeezing the bag when they inspire which helps open the valves, thereby reducing resistance).

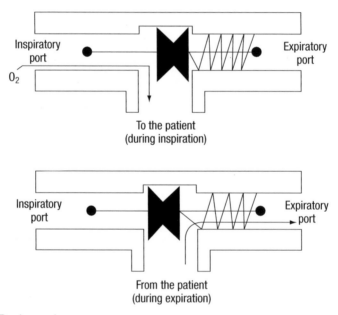

FIGURE 2.39 Reuben valve

Ambu E valve:

➤ This is a double leaf valve.

➤ During positive pressure ventilation, the inspiratory port leaf valve is pushed across and seals the expiratory port, thereby allowing gases to enter the patient.

➤ During expiration, the inspiratory port leaf valve gets pushed back, sealing the inspiratory port while the expiratory port leaf valve gets forced open, allowing exhaled gases to escape into the atmosphere.

➤ During low inspiratory gas flow rates, the inspiratory port leaf valve may not give a good seal across the expiratory port and hence some of the fresh gas can escape across the valve, reducing the fresh gas supply to the patient.

➤ The valve offers resistance and should be used cautiously in the spontaneously
ventilating patient.

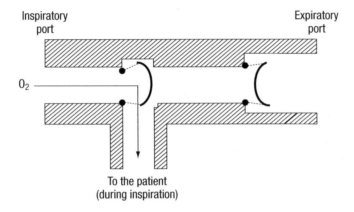

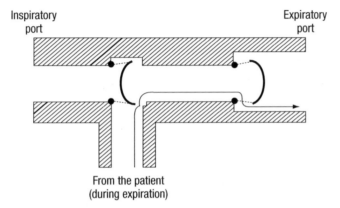

FIGURE 2.40 Ambu E valve

What factors determine the oxygen concentration that can be delivered to the patient?
➤ FiO_2
➤ Oxygen flow rate
➤ Reservoir bag volume (adult size approximately 2600 mL)
➤ Inspiratory flow rate
➤ Respiratory rate
➤ Valve type

CHAPTER 71

Ventilators

How can ventilators be classified?

A question on ventilators will often follow on from a physics question about flow. The simplest way to address this question is to classify ventilation according to the Mapleson classification, which separates it into either 'pressure-generated' or 'flow-generated' ventilation.

A ventilator is a device that delivers gas to the lungs

PRESSURE GENERATOR

- Delivers gas to the patient at a **constant inspiratory pressure** set by the operator

- Usually **time cycled** (i.e. the operator sets the pressure, the number of breaths per minute and the inspiratory:expiratory time ratio and the machine will deliver the breaths accordingly)

- Inspiratory flow rates and tidal volume achieved will depend on the patient's lung compliance (i.e. the stiffer the lungs the lower the resulting tidal volume delivered)

- Risk of barotrauma is low

- Risk of volutrauma is high (so set volume limits)

- The system has some ability to compensate for leaks, as it always delivers a set pressure for a set amount of time

FLOW GENERATOR

- Delivers gas to the patient at a **constant inspiratory flow rate** until it has delivered a pre-set tidal volume

- **Cycles** when the set **tidal volume** has been **delivered**

- Inspiratory pressures reached depend on the patient's lung compliance (i.e. the lower the compliance, the higher the peak inspiratory pressure)

- High risk of barotrauma

- Low risk of volutrauma

- Any leak in the circuit is not compensated for, as the ventilator will perceive that the lost volume has been delivered to the patient

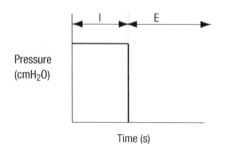

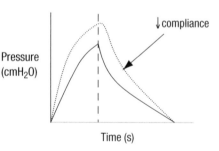

Graphs comparing the pressure profiles of the two different ventilation modes

FIGURE 2.41 Mapleson classification of ventilators

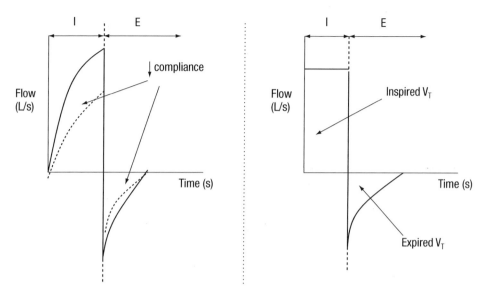

GRAPH 2.42 Comparison of flow profiles for pressure-generated and flow-generated ventilators

A third type of ventilator called the high frequency oscillating ventilator (HFOV) now exists and is being used with increasing frequency on intensive care units.

➤ HFOV employs an 'open lung' strategy, using high PEEP and very small tidal volumes (1–3 mL/kg) at respiratory rates of up to 15 Hz (i.e. 900 breaths per minute!).

➤ It aims to reduce distending pressures in poorly compliant lungs (e.g. in ARDS) and is recommended for those patients requiring a high $FiO_2 > 0.60$ and with high mean airways pressures $> 24\,cmH_2O$.

➤ The mechanism of oxygenation with this type of ventilation is not fully understood, but diffusion, convection and Pendelluft (i.e. movement of gas between different alveolar units with different time constants) are thought to play a part.

DEFINITIONS OF VENTILATORY MODES

CPAP – Continuous Positive Airway Pressure

- A positive pressure (cmH_2O) is applied to the airway of a spontaneously breathing patient via a facial or nasal mask. The pressure is constant through all phases of the ventilatory cycle.
- The positive pressure helps to prevent alveolar and airway closure during expiration and improves lung compliance by moving the lungs up the compliance curve.
- This mode of ventilation is used in the treatment of obstructive sleep apnoea.

PEEP – Positive End Expiratory Pressure

- This is very similar to CPAP, except that it applies to mechanically ventilated patients.
- PEEP is a set level of pressure (cmH_2O) below which the circuit is not allowed to fall at the end of expiration. It is usually set between 5 and 10 cmH_2O.
- It helps to prevent alveolar and airway closure during expiration and improves lung compliance by moving the lungs up the compliance curve.

BiPAP – Bi-level Positive Airway Pressure

- This is a trade name of a particular make of non-invasive ventilators.
- BiPAP is given via a face mask, usually to a conscious and spontaneously ventilating patient.
- The operator sets two levels of pressure; the first is effectively the PEEP, i.e. the level below which the circuit is not allowed to fall. The second is the positive inspiratory pressure, which the ventilator delivers to the patient.
- The machine senses when the patient is taking a breath (via a pressure transducer which senses negative pressure in the system) and then augments their breath to the set pressure. In most cases, cycling is controlled by the machine sensing the patient's respiratory effort. Some models can deliver time cycled positive pressure if the patient fails to make any respiratory effort after a set time has elapsed.

PC – Pressure Control

- Pressure control is used in a mechanically ventilated patient. It is the most basic mode of ventilation.
- The operator sets either the desired tidal volume or desired pressure and the number of breaths per minute and the ventilator will deliver these.
- Any respiratory effort that the patient makes is 'ignored' by the ventilator.

PS – Pressure Support

- Pressure support is used for weaning patients from the ventilator.
- As in BiPAP, the ventilator senses the patient's inspiratory effort and augments it with a pre-set inspiratory pressure.
- It is usual to set two levels of pressure, the principle being the same as that described above for BiPAP.

SIMV – Synchronised Intermittent Mandatory Ventilation

- This mode is a 'half way house' between PC and PS.
- The operator sets the desired tidal volume or inspiratory pressure and the number of breaths per minute. The ventilator will then deliver these breaths.
- However, if the patient makes an inspiratory effort the machine will sense this and augment their breath.

PRVC – Pressure Regulated Volume Control

- In this mode, the operator sets the tidal volume and the machine will deliver this volume in such a way as to give the lowest resultant inspiratory pressure.
- This mode has been developed to try to reduce the risk of barotrauma and to address the issue of different areas of the lung having different compliance in lung diseases such as ARDS.

CHAPTER 72

Lasers

What do you understand by the term 'laser'?
Laser is an acronym for 'light amplification by the stimulated emission of radiation'. Lasers produce an intense beam of light that is monochromatic (single wavelength), coherent (in phase) and collimated (parallel). Laser technology allows high energy intensities to be produced from relatively low power sources.

Describe the basic physics underpinning laser technology
➤ The quantum theory states that electrons are confined to certain energy states but these electrons can move between these energy states depending on whether they absorb or emit energy.
➤ Einstein demonstrated that if you stimulated an atom with a photon of energy, this stimulated atom would in turn emit a photon of equivalent energy, which was in phase with the original stimulating photon. This new emitted photon could now cause a further similar reaction and as such a chain reaction and hence amplification of the system would ensue.
➤ In lasers, an external source of energy (e.g. high voltage or flash of light) is applied to a laser medium.
➤ This increases the energy state of the electrons within the laser medium and moves them up from a 'ground' energy state to an 'excited' energy state.
➤ When these excited electrons return to their original ground state they emit energy in the form of light or radiation.
➤ This emitted energy can then stimulate further electrons within the medium, thereby amplifying the whole process.
➤ The wavelength of light produced depends on the lasing medium that is used.

What are the fundamental components within a laser device?
➤ External energy source (to 'stimulate' the electrons)
➤ Laser medium (this can be a solid, liquid or a gas)
➤ Chamber containing the laser medium
➤ System of mirrors (to allow 'amplification' of radiation)
➤ A partially reflective mirror (to allow the emitted radiation to exit the system)
➤ Windows at each end of the device are inclined to Brewster's angle (this is the angle of incidence at which light is perfectly transmitted with no reflection, thereby ensuring that 100% of the light is transmitted through the windows)
➤ Fibre-optic cable (to direct the laser beam)

List the different types of lasers with their clinical applications?
➤ **Nd-YAG (neodymium-doped-yttrium aluminium garnet) lasers**
  • Crystal used as a lasing medium in solid-state lasers.
  • Wavelength of light produced is 1064 nm (near infrared region).
  • Good tissue penetration (as it is not absorbed by water).
  • Used typically for endoscopic surgery (there have been reports of inadvertent

pneumathoraces during ENT surgery due to these lasers penetrating and affecting tissues deeper than anticipated).
➤ **Carbon dioxide lasers**
  ● Used as a lasing medium in gas-state lasers.
  ● Highest power laser currently available (also used in industry for cutting, welding and engraving).
  ● Wavelength of light produced is 10.6 μm (infrared region).
  ● Poor tissue penetration of < 200 μm (as it is absorbed by water causing it to vaporise and destroy tissue contents).
  ● Used typically for superficial surgery (e.g. dermabrasion and laser 'facelifts').
  ● Unsuitable for endoscopic use.
➤ **Argon lasers**
  ● Used as a lasing medium in gas-state lasers.
  ● Wavelength of light produced is between 400 and 700 nm (blue-green region of the visible spectrum).
  ● Good penetration through transparent tissues (e.g. aqueous humour, vitreous humour and lens of the eye).
  ● Maximally absorbed by red-pigmented tissues (e.g. birth marks, haemoglobin).
  ● Used typically in eye surgery (e.g. retinal phototherapy) and in dermatological procedures to cosmetically enhance pigmented lesions.
➤ **Dye lasers**
  ● Organic dye used as a lasing medium in liquid-state lasers.
  ● Wavelength of light produced is broad and varies occurring to the dye used.
  ● Used typically in 'beauty clinics' to even out skin tone.

How are lasers classified?
➤ **Class 1** – power does not exceed maximum permissible exposure for the eye.
➤ **Class 2** – power up to 1 mW and visible laser beams only. Eye protected by blink reflex.
➤ **Class 3a** – power up to 5 mW and visible spectrum only but now laser beam must be expanded (so that maximum irradiance does not exceed $25\,W/m^2$). Eyes protected by blink reflex.
➤ **Class 3b** – power up to 0.5 W and any wavelength. Direct viewing hazardous. Eye protection essential.
➤ **Class 4** – power > 0.5 W and any wavelength. Extremely hazardous and capable of igniting inflammable materials. Eye protection essential.

What are the hazards of laser surgery?
Lasers are hazardous to use because they combine high energy intensities confined within a small spot size (i.e. very concentrated) and transmitted in a non-divergent beam (i.e. these devices do not lose power with increasing distance from the laser source). For comparison, when looking directly into sunlight the eye is exposed to approximately $150\,W/m^2$ but if inadvertently looking into a laser beam, the eye is exposed to approximately $3 \times 10^6\,W/m^2$!
➤ **Environment:**
  ● Fire and explosions – flammable spirits, oxygen and nitrous oxide can get collected in the drapes and these can get ignited if the laser beam is directed to it.
➤ **Staff:**
  ● Eyes – if the laser beam hits the retina, a permanent blind spot can develop but if it hits the optic nerve permanent blindness can be caused (CO_2 lasers do not penetrate the cornea and therefore cannot affect the retina).

- Skin – if the laser beam hits the skin, a burning sensation is felt and this will trigger self-protecting manoeuvres.
➤ **Laser hazards affecting the anaesthetised patient:**
  - Eyes – as above
  - Skin – now self-protecting manoeuvres do not come to play and therefore patients are at risk of laser burns.
  - Airway fire – this is a real risk during laser surgery to the upper airway (this is an anaesthetic emergency and therefore you must be well versed with both the precautions needed to prevent this and the immediate management required to deal with this).

What precautions are taken to minimise the hazards of laser surgery?
➤ **General:**
  - Designated laser protection supervisor for each theatre.
  - Staff all trained and educated in laser use.
  - Doors locked, windows closed and signs displayed to protect those outside theatre.
➤ **Equipment:**
  - Eye protection goggles (laser beam wavelength-specific) for both staff and patient.
  - Surgical instruments with a black or matt finish to minimise refection of laser beam.
➤ **Anaesthetic considerations for upper airway laser surgery:**
  - Double-cuffed, laser-resistant endotracheal tube (these are often flexible stainless steel tubes with two cuffs to ensure a tracheal seal if the upper cuff is accidentally damaged by the laser).
  - Cuffs filled with saline (air-filled cuffs may ignite if hit by the laser).
  - Throat packed with wet swabs (to protect adjacent areas from inadvertent laser burns).
  - Oxygen – air mix (as nitrous oxide is more flammable).
  - $FiO_2 < 0.25$ if tolerated.

What are the basic concepts in managing an airway fire?
➤ Call for help and inform your immediate theatre team.
➤ Surgeon to switch off laser and flood the operation site with water.
➤ Disconnect the anaesthetic machine.
➤ Remove endotracheal tube if feasible (remember that even laser-resistant tubes can ignite).
➤ Ventilate the patient with a bag-valve-mask circuit (if necessary continue anaesthesia with TIVA).
➤ Surgeon to inspect the airway with rigid bronchoscope.
➤ Refer to ITU (airway fires can cause significant lung injury and ARDS – patient may require ventilation, dexamethasone, and humidified oxygen).

CHAPTER 73

Ultrasound

What are the clinical uses of ultrasound?
In the last decade there has been a rapid expansion in the use of ultrasound within anaesthetics and critical care medicine. Use of ultrasound has become routine in the theatre environment to aid vascular line insertion (NICE 2002), guide peripheral nerve blockade, e.g. interscalene nerve blocks (NICE 2009), and in some centres to also guide catheter placement within the epidural space (NICE 2008). In the critical care setting, ultrasound is routinely used for vascular line insertion, cardiac output monitoring, echocardiography, transcranial Doppler, pleural aspiration, ascitic drainage, assessment of hepatic portal vein flow and detection of venous thromboembolism.

What are the principles of ultrasound?
➤ Ultrasound is an imaging modality that utilises high frequency sound waves (in the region of 2 MHz) in order to image structures within the body.
➤ Ultrasound waves are generated by applying an electric field to a piezoelectric crystal in the transducer, which leads to the crystal vibrating and generating ultrasound waves.
➤ Four different modes of ultrasound are utilised in medical imaging:
  • **A Mode** – a single transducer scans a line through the body with the echoes plotted on the screen as a function of depth
  • **B Mode** – a linear array of transducers simultaneously scans a plane through the body allowing it to be viewed as a two-dimensional image
  • **M ('Motion') Mode** – a rapid sequence of B mode scans produces sequential images
  • **Doppler Mode** – utilises the Doppler principle to enable detection and velocity of flow
➤ Tissues within the body differ in their ability to transmit sound waves.
➤ When the sound wave encounters a change in tissue, part of the sound wave is transmitted and part is reflected back to the transducer. It is the reflected sound waves that are converted into an image. The time taken for the sound waves to return to the transducer provides an indication of the depth of the tissue interface.
➤ Ultrasound gel is essential to acquire good images, acting as a coupling medium, which reduces the attenuation of the ultrasound waveform.
➤ B-Mode is the commonest method of displaying the ultrasound image. Here the intensity of the echoes reflected back to the transducer is proportional to the whitening of the film. Thus structures with no internal echoes appear black (anechoic) whereas structures containing internal echoes appear white (echogenic).
➤ Ultrasound is good for examining fluid filled structures (e.g. vessels) and soft tissues but not for air containing structures (e.g. lung tissue) or for calcium rich structures (e.g. bone).
➤ Advantages of ultrasound as an imaging modality: relatively inexpensive, widely available, non-invasive and no ionising radiation therefore safe in children and pregnancy.

➤ Disadvantages of ultrasound as an imaging modality: operator dependent, cannot be used to image lung or bone, resolution of the ultrasound image is inversely proportional to the depth of penetration and so it is not good for examining deep structures or imaging obese patients.

➤ Doppler ultrasound is based upon the Doppler principle – sound waves reflected from a moving target (e.g. red blood cells) have a different frequency from the incident sound wave. This frequency shift is proportional to the velocity of the flowing blood. Doppler allows not only the detection of flowing blood but also enables its velocity to be quantified.

➤ Doppler ultrasound can be colour coded and superimposed on to a real time B-mode image to indicate the direction of blood flow. BART – blue indicates flow 'away' from the ultrasound probe and red 'towards' the probe.

Give a clinical example of a device utilising ultrasound

➤ **Transoesophageal Doppler**
  - This has now become established as a relatively non-invasive method of cardiac output monitoring.
  - Doppler probe is positioned in the mid-oesophagus in order to measure red blood cell velocity in the descending thoracic aorta.
  - Aortic cross-sectional area is estimated from a nomogram (age/height/weight) or in some devices it is measured.
  - Once the probe is positioned correctly, it utilises the Doppler principle to measure red blood cell velocity from which blood flow can then be calculated.

CHAPTER 74

CT and MRI

A transfer to the CT or MRI scanner with an anaesthetised patient is not a task to be undertaken lightly. There is good reason that the CT scanner is affectionately known as the 'doughnut of death'. When answering a question on scan transfers, it is important to show the examiners that you are well prepared to cope with the potential pitfalls that may occur on your journey.

What are the principles behind computed tomography (CT) scanning?

The name comes from the Greek 'tomo', meaning slice and 'graphein', to write. CTs take a series of X-ray images around a central axis, either in a discontinuous 'shoot and step' process, or in a continuous 'spiral' fashion. The latter are much quicker and so may reduce motion artefact, and enable better 3D reconstruction of images.

What are the principles behind magnetic resonance imaging (MRI)?

➤ MRI is an alternative way of producing images of the body.
➤ MRI visualises soft tissues much better than does CT, and therefore is more useful in the study of the brain, spinal cord and musculoskeletal system.
➤ Atoms with unpaired electrons or protons are in a state of spin that can be affected by the application of an external magnetic field.
➤ Hydrogen ions found in water and fat molecules (which make up 60–70% of the body) are affected in this way and so, when the patient enters the powerful magnetic field of the scanner (1–2 tesla), their protons align in the direction of the field.
➤ The protons then begin to resonate at their 'precision frequency'.
➤ The powerful magnet is called the 'primary magnet' and its magnetic field is generated by an electrical current passing through coils of wire, which are cooled with liquid helium.
➤ Once the atoms have lined up, a radiofrequency coil is turned on, generating a second current at right angles to the first.
➤ The energy generated by this coil is absorbed by the hydrogen ions and disrupts their alignment.
➤ When the radiofrequency coil is turned off, the protons release energy (in the form of low frequency radiation) and return to their original position.
➤ It is this low frequency radiation that is detected by the scanner, and reconstructed into images.
➤ Different tissues will give out different amounts of energy and return to their equilibrium position at different rates, allowing for differentiation between them. This exchange of energy between spin states is called 'resonance'.
➤ Another component of the MRI scanner is the 'gradient magnet'. These are smaller magnets that are applied to allow fine-tuning and focusing of the image on the area being studied. The banging noise in the MRI is the sound of these magnets being turned on and off.
➤ MRIs are either T1 or T2 weighted and this refers to the amount of time elapsed

between the radiofrequency magnet being switched off and the image being taken, i.e. the 'relaxation time'. T1 images are taken earlier than T2. In T1 images fat is bright and water is black, in T2 images fat is black and water is bright.
➤ The entire scanner is housed in a room lined with copper or aluminium, and this room is referred to as the Faraday cage.

What are the indications for general anaesthesia in the scanner?
➤ Unstable patient (e.g. for airway protection or from ITU)
➤ Young child if they cannot co-operate and lie still
➤ Patient with learning difficulties, as above
➤ Very anxious or claustrophobic patient
➤ Patients with movement disorders or who are unable to lie still for sufficiently long.

What are the problems associated with anaesthesia in the scanning department?
➤ Generic problems:
  • **Patients are removed to an often remote and isolated area:** This area may be unfamiliar to the responsible doctor. It is important, therefore, to consider who will be available to help should there be an emergency during the trip and if possible, to familiarise oneself with the department and the equipment available there before the transfer.
  • **Cold and noisy environment:** Ambient temperature in an MRI scanner is cool in order to prevent the magnet from overheating. The magnets produce a lot of noise and earplugs must therefore be used and patients covered in order to minimise risk of hypothermia.
  • **Claustrophobic environment:** Space within scanners is extremely limited, more so in the MRI scanner and some patients can find this very distressing.
  • **Limited space for anaesthetic equipment**
  • **Limited access to the patient:** Once the patient is in the scanner it can be practically impossible to get to them. Before the scan begins it is important to satisfy yourself that all the leads reach far enough, that the patient is stable and that you can see the monitor. The scan may take some time, especially if it is an MRI.
➤ **Specific problems related to the MRI scanner:** The magnet in the MRI adds a whole new layer of problems.
  • **Ferrous implants:** Within the magnetic field, ferrous implants (e.g. pacemakers, defibrillators, cochlear implants, some aneurysm clips and foreign bodies) are prone to displacement or torque forces, which can lead to serious patient injury. These patients must not enter the MRI scanner. Non-ferrous implants are prone to heating and patients must be warned of this. Both types of implants can cause image artefacts.
  • **Ferrous equipment:** Ferrous-containing equipment like laryngoscopes, stethoscopes, pagers, and gas cylinders are prone to significant movement within the 50G line and should therefore not be taken beyond this point unless securely fastened. Magnetic strips on identity badges and credit cards will also be wiped if taken within the magnetic field. Ideally, only 'MR safe' and 'MR conditional' equipment should be used within the scanner.
  • **Monitoring:** Special 'MR safe' ECG electrodes, BP cuffs and pulse oximeters are required. ECG leads are short and plaited to minimise the risk of magnetically induced currents within them, which can burn the patient (burns are the commonest MRI-associated injury). If a standard anaesthetic machine is used, this is housed outside the Faraday cage with an extra long Bain circuit connecting

it to the patient. Long gas analysis sampling lines cause a delay in monitoring. Monitoring equipment can introduce stray radiofrequency currents, which can degrade the image quality.

- **Delivery of anaesthesia:** 'MR conditional' infusion pumps should ideally be used. However, standard pumps can also be used outside the 100G. Volatile agents can be administered using a 'MR conditional' anaesthetic machine. If this is not available, a standard anaesthetic machine can be used outside of the cage with an extra-long Bain circuit.

How are items to be used within an MRI scanner classified?

The ASTM International and FDA have recently proposed new terminology for all items and equipment being used in the MR environment (the term 'MR compatible' is no longer suitable):

- ➤ **MR Safe:** Items are completely free of all metallic components. They are non-metallic, non-conductive and non-radiofrequency reactive. They pose no hazards in any MR environment.
- ➤ **MR Conditional:** Items are safe under certain tested magnetic conditions, which should be enumerated on the product (i.e. the magnetic field strength in which the product can be safely used is stated).
- ➤ **MR Unsafe:** Items pose a hazard in any MR environment.

What is the standard international unit of magnetic strength?

- ➤ SI unit for magnetic flux is the weber (Wb)
- ➤ SI unit for magnetic flux density is the tesla (T), which is used for large densities. For smaller densities a smaller unit the gauss (G) is used. An average MR scanner produces between 1–1.5 T (although newer machines can now generate up to 3–5 T), while earth's magnetic field is about 1G.

$$1T = 1\,Wb/m^2$$
$$1T = 10,000\ gauss$$

Index